The
Empowered
Patient

Dr. Julia Hallisy

The Empowered Patient ©2008 Julia A. Hallisy, D.D.S.

Theempoweredpatient.com
PatientsafetyCA.org
595 Buckingham Way, Suite # 305
San Francisco, CA 94132

To order visit TheEmpoweredPatient.com

Cover design: George Foster, www.fostercovers.com
Interior design & typesetting: Liz Tufte, www.folio-bookworks.com
Indexing: Galen L. Schroeder, Dakota Indexing

ISBN: 978-0-6151-7791-5

Disclaimer

This book was written to educate and inform the reader about the specific skills they need and action steps they can take to ensure that they receive safe, high-quality medical care. *The Empowered Patient* is intended to be a catalyst for individuals to cultivate mutually respectful relationships with their healthcare providers, to learn to ask the right questions, and to communicate effectively about their treatment options and outcomes. It is informational in nature and is not intended as a substitute for professional medical advice.

Acknowledgements

I am indebted to a number of people who shared their time, expertise or proofreading skills: John Hallisy, Sonia Bajone, Susan Imperial, Steve Pomerantz, Tony Seba, Kathy Murphy, R.N., Shauna Lobre, R.N., Helen Haskell, Jennifer Dingman, Catherine Reuter-Lake, Herb Bielawa and Peter Van Zandt, J.D.

Special thanks to my editor, Amanita Rosenbush, who was part of this project from the beginning. I am especially grateful for her patience while working with a novice and for helping me think and feel like a writer.

To my agent, Jim Cypher, for his belief in this book and for his tireless efforts in the quest for publication.

To Liz Tufte and George Foster for their work designing the interior and the cover of the book.

To my husband, John Hallisy, and to our sons, Daniel and Kevin, for sharing my vision and helping me fulfill my promise to Kate to write this book.

Dedication

To my loving husband, John Hallisy, I have no doubt that we were meant to be parents to the wondrous being that was Kate and to stand beside each other as we followed and supported her down the path her life was destined to take.

To my mother, Sonia Bajone, who is a constant source of support and the one who taught me that you can survive the loss of a child with dignity and grace.

To my sons, Daniel Hallisy and Kevin Hallisy, who gave me a reason to go on and who showed me that I could still have joy in my life.

And, most of all, to my beloved daughter, Katherine Hallisy. You asked me once if you would have to wait long in Heaven before seeing us again. Now I know that my answer was true. The time only seems long to those left behind.

Contents

Chapter One

Introduction

Of all the millions of people who interact with our health care system every year, only a fraction is even vaguely aware of the number of errors that occur or the risk of harm that is present.

We are somewhat educated by the few incidents of medical error that appear in the media. "Dateline NBC," for example, began 2002 with a report on a routine ear surgery at Martin Memorial Hospital in Stuart, Florida. The patient, a seven-year-old boy named Ben Kolb died after liquid adrenalin, instead of the anesthetic lidocaine, was mistakenly injected into him. The source of the problem? Both drugs, which look identical, were in open cups next to each other on the surgeon's tray and were mislabeled. At Beth Israel Hospital in New York, 30-year-old Lisa Smart lost her life during a simple outpatient surgery for a uterine fibroid. The surgeon was using a new piece of equipment for the first time and had a sales rep in the operating room to guide him. The results were tragic: Mrs. Smart died when her heart and lungs gave out because of a massive overload of saline solution. In 1993, 39-year-old Denise DeSoto went into a coma following hand surgery at a major medical center in California. During surgery, Mrs. DeSoto's breathing was not monitored closely enough and mucus obstructed her breathing tube and deprived her brain of oxygen. None of these people entered the hospital believing that they were undergoing life-threatening procedures. If anything, they thought their treatment would be fairly routine.

Some of us are aware of these problems because of news reports, and some know people personally who have endured medical mishaps. There are also people, of course, who have even been through it themselves. We keep waiting for legislators to come to our rescue, or for insurance companies, doctors and hospitals to put an end to the momentous mistakes that threaten people's lives. There have been attempts in individual institutions and by local and national organizations to rectify the problem, but the efforts have yet to make a significant impact on the enormity of the predicament.

No one is immune. The people in the stories above all went in for procedures they believed to be ordinary and uneventful; some never left the hospital. Fatalities are brought about by numerous sources. Nosocomial infection (hospital-acquired) accounts for 90,000 deaths a year in the United States, a number greater than all other accidental deaths. Adverse drug reactions are responsible for as many as 100,000 fatalities a year, making it another leading cause of death. To err on the side of fairness, we should take into account the complaints of critics who dispute these figures. Let's be magnanimous and divide the numbers in half. We can still extrapolate to meaning that as many as 95,000 people die each year in a country that has the most technologically advanced medical delivery system in the world, not to mention the most expensive. And now, tragically, we have a hideous new point of reference for these figures. The number of lives lost to medical error is roughly equivalent to a World Trade Center attack occurring every two weeks during the year. And while the entire nation mourned our identifiable victims and heroes, the victims of medical mishap are mourned silently and individually. Yet they are heroes nonetheless in a virtually unknown war. We don't see their pictures, we don't know their names, and there are no medals awarded for their sacrifices.

The media and the government do try to warn us against the dangers we are up against with admonitions such as, "Make sure all your healthcare providers wash their hands before touching you," or "Don't sign blanket consent forms," or "Check your medication to be sure your pharmacy did not make any mistakes," or "Don't forget to tell the hospital to assign you an RN and not a lesser trained nurses aide," or the all-inclusive mantra, "Be sure to include yourself as a member of your team." Good advice, but what *exactly* are you supposed to do to ensure that these things actually happen? Many of you who are reading this right now don't know that you have a right to customize your consent form. You do not know the correct name of your medication from reading your prescription. You don't know whom to ask in advance to secure a highly qualified RN. It certainly should be obvious to everyone who works in a hospital or a doctor's office that they should be washing their hands on a regular basis, but how can you make sure they do? We cannot sit back and assume that someone else is looking out for our interests; we can and should be doing these things for ourselves.

Many of the issues I will be covering in this book apply to you whether you are going to the hospital for a "routine" procedure (let's face it, anything that is invasive to your body is hardly routine) or whether you're rushed in from a 3-car pile-up on I-80. In my case, I was embroiled in the medical system for years because my daughter, Katherine Eileen Hallisy, was diagnosed when she was five months old with an aggressive eye cancer called bilateral retinoblastoma. Kate's decade-long plan of treatment included experiences with radiation, chemotherapy, reconstructive surgeries, the removal of her right eye, a hospital-acquired infection that led to toxic shock syndrome, and an above-the-knee amputation. During all those years of interacting with physicians and hospitals, I encountered virtually every problem a patient and their loved ones can face. In this book, I will use the knowledge gained from my own experiences, as well as those of other patients, to point out the hidden dangers that are inherent in our medical delivery system. Your need to feel safe is not self-indulgent.

You have a right to expect a reasonable degree of safety. In fact, where else should you expect to be safer than in a hospital?

My husband and I spent years of our lives in hospital hallways, waiting rooms and emergency rooms. We have spoken to hundreds of patients, family members, nurses, and physicians. The common denominator among all is that the parties involved had their own unique disappointments and frustrations with the system. This marks the eighteenth year since my initiation into it, and I can assure you that progress is painfully slow. Insurance reimbursements to hospitals have not kept up with their cost of doing business; to reduce overhead, staffing levels at healthcare facilities have been brought to dangerously low levels; the compliance rates with infection control measures such as hand washing are not where they need to be; and the morale of healthcare workers is suffering.

In short, our healthcare system is still frustrating, dangerous, and fraught with errors. The efforts of legislators and patient advocacy groups to combat the problems only show us that it may be years before there is a legal path out of the dilemma. For six long years, lawmakers in California worked on passing a federal Patients' Bill of Rights. To date, it is still in legislative purgatory. It has currently been shelved until someone finds the courage to bring it before the legislature yet again. In the meantime, what are patients supposed to do? Are we to continue to sit idly by while others argue the issues? It is my hope that the public makes it clear that we are no longer willing to risk our health while lawmakers bandy ideas and debate picayune points instead of working together to find solutions.

Fortunately, the public is beginning to be aware of the dangers as a result of the media coverage of newsworthy stories and because of a mandate directly from the Clinton White House in 2000 to reduce medical error by 50 percent over a five-year period. Startling statistics and reports of the thousands of errors and patient injuries have systematically exposed the potentially deadly deficiencies in our medical delivery system. In December 2006 the Institute for Healthcare Improvement launched a campaign to reduce hospital injuries by 5 million over the next two years. *5 million!* These efforts have served to put the public on guard, but unfortunately they are no guarantee of meaningful legislative or widespread, mandatory systematic changes. This means that it is often left to the individual to work out a plan to keep him or herself safe.

While it appears on the surface that people who are struggling with illness should not have to shoulder the responsibility for ensuring safe care, the reality is that patients today and their advocates must step up to the plate. They must be informed, proactive and vocal about demanding proper care. Once enough patients know what they have a right to expect and diplomatically, yet effectively, ask for it, it will be impossible for the industry to ignore their demands.

At the present time, the powers-that-be in our society do not believe that the average person is willing to take on this task. They don't believe people will expend the effort to educate themselves about healthcare issues or to take responsibility for the quality of the care they receive. I hope we will prove them wrong. High expectations, however, do not mean unreasonable expectations. Most people are smart enough to comprehend the fact that there is no such thing as absolutely risk-free care or guaranteed cures. They know when they see their doctor or enter the hospital, they will not automatically return home with a clean bill of health. Some conditions are still unalterable, some injuries still inoperable, some diseases are incurable, and some maladies are with us for life. Our bodies are inherently vulnerable to disease, accidents, sickness and death. But given the inevitability of all this, we still have a right to expect safe, low-risk care, especially since our per capita healthcare expenditures are the highest in the world.

My Message

My husband and I became more savvy and educated the longer my daughter's illness went on. As we progressed, we slowly came to realize that the quality of healthcare she was receiving, as mediocre as it sometimes was, was actually far superior to the care other families around us in the hospital were receiving. They began to notice this discrepancy as well, and they wanted to know how we knew the things we did and who had given us such valuable "inside" information. We had to explain to them that we had come across everything we knew the hard way—by watching our daughter suffer through medical errors, misdiagnoses and inexperienced medical providers, and investigating the mistakes and taking steps to make sure that they didn't occur again. The experiences made us vow to find answers and solutions so that if we ever had to go through a health crisis again, we would be prepared.

While we were customizing our solutions to the problems that were right in front of us, we soon realized that the general principles we were applying were universal. They would work for anyone, regardless of the diagnosis or the person's degree of medical knowledge. The reason for this is that all of these problems are the result of flaws in the medical system itself, and the system works pretty much the same way no matter which hospital one is in and no matter what medical condition one is contending with. The system is the system. Once you, the reader, understand what your particular problem areas are likely to be within the system, you can prepare your tool kit ahead of time.

By looking beneath the surface, it was easy to recognize that the issues my family confronted were fundamental. Everyone entering the system will deal with some variation of the same issues. It doesn't matter if patients are having open heart surgery or a simple tonsillectomy, they may still have to contend with infection, inexperience, privacy violations, ignored complaints, complete strangers performing invasive procedures on their bodies and surgical procedures that could go beyond the scope of what they thought they were authorizing. My family had to confront every one of these, and the odds are that if you enter America's medical system, you will stumble into at least one of these before too long.

To interact competently with the medical establishment, you

do not need to be a professional or have a Ph.D. It is the purpose of this book to arm each and every reader with the information he needs to ensure the best healthcare possible. All the recommendations included here can be easily implemented by people who have no medical training whatsoever, by those who feel intimidated by physicians, and even by those individuals who have never been to a hospital except, perhaps, to be born. What patients and their loved ones have never been told, and what is my mission to convey, is that there are many simple actions they can take to keep themselves safe and protect their rights as consumers. And that is why I titled this book *The Empowered Patient*. You can do this for yourself; it isn't brain surgery.

But before you can become strong and capable, you must first understand the ways in which you are vulnerable. You must identify the problem areas that you are likely to encounter so that you can formulate effective strategies in advance. You have to be alerted to the areas of risk and then acquire the specific skills you need to reduce the odds of being harmed in the course of your medical care. The salient message of this book is that those who are knowledgeable about a subject are better able to assess information being presented to them by professionals, they are prepared to recognize potential hazards before they show up on the front doorstep, and they are primed to take decisive steps once they have identified any problems. In addition, consumers who possess a higher level of understanding about the medical system and how it works will also have higher expectations about the quality of care they are entitled to and the level of safety they should demand. If the patients of today were armed with the right information, they could unite as the largest, most cost-effective and most powerful grass roots lobbying group in history. Medical patients already possess strength in numbers. They just haven't put their extraordinary power to the test.

The statistics reflecting the somber and startling reality of just how high-risk an endeavor it is to enter a hospital can be overwhelming. It can make anyone feel helpless. The reality, however, is that you can have a powerful, even life-saving influence on your healing process or on that of a loved one. My husband and I struggled to find our way through the complex medical maze, and when the system failed us, we had to find our own solutions. It is my fervent hope that you can learn from our solutions. The information presented in this book came at a high price physically, economically and emotionally. But now I possess the knowledge and the responsibility to help other patients reduce their chances of injury, cut down on the risk of errors, understand the danger of miscommunications and lessen the instances of personal frustration and anger. I want this journey to be far easier for those coming up behind us.

The Empowered Patient will arm readers with the knowledge they need to claim a voice in and authority over their health care. The public will finally be able to view their relationships with healthcare providers as partnerships and to see themselves for the first time as researchers, investigators, and decision-makers. The adage, "If you're not part of the solution, then you are part of the problem" applies here. In short, empowered patients are those who are both informed and willing to accept the responsibility of self-directed medical care.

Chapter Two

Your Healthcare Team

Thirty years ago, if you were afflicted with heart and kidney problems, your practitioner, the only one you had, would have been expected to consider a variety of complicated diagnoses and then competently manage every component of your care. The practice of medicine at that time typically involved one individual who provided comprehensive care for a wide range of conditions. Since then, medicine has become a six-headed monster because the amount of information available about the diagnosis and treatment of illness has increased exponentially, and no one person can possibly master the data on every ailment afflicting the human body. Modern medicine has evolved to the point where no one is expected to be an expert at everything. The inevitable outcome of this inundation? The trend toward specialization. The management of the complex, multi-faceted needs of an individual by a team of experts poses obvious benefits to patients, yet it can easily become a liability if the members of the team don't check in with each other, and in fact, if they function only as a loose collection of people who *happen to be* caring for the same person.

A modern healthcare team necessitates the collaboration of a number of individuals, each of whom possesses knowledge, ideas, resources and experience that ought to be applied, in tandem, to the specific needs of patients. A good analogy here is a sports team. In a successful franchise, each member excels at what he or she does. The team as a whole possesses a common identity and goals. Members practice together, learn the same plays, and consistently review their own performance to see what works and what doesn't. Imagine the outcome, however, if individual basketball players strategize only for themselves or if they ran down the court and "winged" it on every play. Without focusing on one joint goal, without well-rehearsed strategies for passing, rebounding, and shooting, the game would quickly disintegrate into chaos. And the outcome? They would lose the game. Apply this same principle to medicine. A patient is admitted for a heart bypass procedure. She is attended by a surgeon, a cardiologist, nurses, pharmacists, nutritionists, and therapists (to aid in lifestyle changes such as reducing stress levels). They all form their own picture of what is wrong with the woman and what she needs, but they don't always coordinate the information. In a hospital, where the stakes are so much higher than at a sports coliseum, the odds of all of the above sitting down every day in one room and developing a detailed, comprehensive plan for the patient's treatment, recovery, evaluation of therapeutic success, as well as being dedicated to their own ongoing communication as a team, are small. At the peril of all of us, hospitals don't often operate that way.

Yet the team approach is a practical necessity in response to the realities of modern medical practice. Doctors in private practice may see 30 to 40 people a day in their office; they don't have a great deal of time for overseeing hospital stays. The number of physicians who are able to juggle demanding in-office primary care as well as high tech in-patient hospital medicine is rapidly declining. Consequently, physicians with private practices increasingly rely on hospital physicians to care for their patients once they check in. The forms you sign when you are admitted might have your primary care doctor's name at the top, and your wristband and chart will contain his or her name. However, don't let that lull you into a false sense of security that the doctor you have been seeing for years will be directing and overseeing your care during your hospital stay, even if from a distance. In most institutions, nothing could be further from the truth. Once the patient enters those giant glass doors, a shift of power takes place, and those who are not aware of the shift will be confused, disappointed, and angry at a time when they ought to be channeling all their personal resources toward one goal: getting well. Once you are admitted, your personal physician disappears, and what appears in her place is a team. Even in an emergency — when most people have a particularly keen interest in their own physician overseeing their case — it is unlikely that this will occur. Many private doctors now form large on-call groups to cover all the emergencies that are bound to occur for such a huge number of patients. Each doctor might be on call only one night a month, so the odds of it being your doctor in a given emergency are small. This puts the burden on patients and their loved ones to form immediate working relationships with virtual strangers at a time when they are particularly vulnerable.

Yes, physicians still care about their patients, but the level of personal interest and concern many have come to expect by watching doctor shows on TV is pure illusion. You may have grown up watching the intimate bedside manner of Marcus Welby, M.D., and think your doctor will show up in your hospital room and share charming anecdotes with you. Or, if you're of this generation, you might admire the dedication of the physicians on the television show "ER" who track their patients down after hours to provide them with medications they've paid for with their own money. But this level of involvement comes straight out of the imagination of screenwriters. It is rare for doctors to spend more than a few minutes at their patient's bedside, and we certainly can't expect them to pay the pharmacy bill out of their own pockets. The prevalence of large on-call groups means that a doctor might respond personally to a patient's after-hours emergencies, but it may only be one night every few weeks.

At some point in your life, no matter how healthy you are, hospitalization will probably be inevitable. You and your advocates need to understand the role each team member will play in the intricate synchronization that modern hospital care now requires. Basic knowledge of their duties and the level of care you should expect from each person is the crucial first step; it will allow you to assume your rightful place at the center of your healthcare team. Don't start out of the gate a length behind everyone else, putting yourself in the position of having to come from behind. Investing a small amount of time to acquaint yourself with the players right at the start will let you be an empowered patient, and it will also help you use the information presented in this book to its full potential. It means you will not only ask the right question, but you'll ask it of the right person.

So who are these people who take over the minute you enter the hospital? The following sections describe the members of the medical team and explain what roles they play.

HOUSE STAFF is a generalized term used by the hospital to cover interns, residents and fellows. These people are not fully autonomous doctors yet, but are still in the process of completing their respective training programs. The hospital employs them to provide both initial and ongoing medical care to patients. Remember that these individuals may sound knowledgeable at your bedside, but they haven't finished all their hands-on training requirements yet. They are, in fact, still students with varying levels of experience and expertise. As such, house staff doctors are under the supervision of members of the more senior medical staff.

House staff is responsible for duties such as assessing a patient's medical history, evaluating the chief complaint, formulating a treatment plan and writing orders, coordinating consultations, assisting with medical procedures, and supervising and teaching other students.

In many institutions, when patients enter a hospital (especially a teaching hospital), they immediately become the responsibility of the house staff. Even if your personal physician *is* managing your hospital care, the house staff will probably be in control of it at some juncture, for instance in the evenings, on weekends, or in the event of an emergency when your personal physician isn't available. Your normally "hands-on" physician is bound to be unavailable at some time, at which point you may discover that the office colleague who is covering for him routinely defers to the house staff at the hospital for all after-hours medical decisions.

You may assume that the execution of your doctor's plan is a foregone conclusion, but it could actually be abandoned on the spur of the moment because of lab test results, x-ray readings, or just personal preferences of a resident. Your personal physician may write orders and communicate his plan to you, but that plan isn't written in stone. Members of the house staff, even those with far less medical experience, *have the authority to alter your physician's orders*. A completely different course of treatment could be deemed superior by the house staff.

I was faced with this situation years ago. Our own oncologist had ordered morphine for my daughter. I was nervous about using such a strong narcotic on a child, but he assured me that it was the only way to keep her comfortable, and so I agreed. Then a first-year resident, who was in charge of the unit for the weekend, apparently with the same reservations I had had, downgraded the medication to Tylenol. Because Kate was receiving a particularly noxious type of chemotherapy that caused vicious sores all through her esophagus, the change placed her in far more pain that a little dose of liquid Tylenol would ever handle. Not only was the dose inadequate for the pain, but Kate could not swallow the Tylenol. As soon as the nurse informed me that the order had been changed, I attempted to contact my daughter's private physician. But he was unavailable for the weekend, and I was referred back to the very resident who had changed the order in the first place! A battle, of sorts, ensued before the order for morphine could be reinstated. This kind of occurrence throws people for a loop. Patients sit there in their flimsy hospital gowns feeling exposed and powerless; they are panicked about the changes they had no hand in making. The house staff is five steps ahead of them, and they're left to wonder what just happened.

Patients do not have to be left out of the loop. A prototype for including patients in their own care was initiated by Concord Hospital in Concord, New Hampshire. This institution has a new vision for conducting rounds (often the only point in the day when patients have contact with their team) in their cardiac unit. Instead of dropping by on an individual basis, Concord's doctors make an effort to come in the room together. This means that all the decision-makers are in the same place at the same time—right in front of the patient. The patient is able to see a coordinated, overall plan of treatment instead of trying to piece it together for herself based on snippets of conversation throughout the day. The policy is to try to inform the patient what time of day this event will occur so the person can have her family or advocate there for the meeting. Members of the team also strive to use "ordinary language instead of medical terminology." Rounds begins with a review of the previous day's plan, and each member can offer feedback about what might have gone right or wrong the day before. Only then is the plan for the current day developed, clarified, and then summarized for the patient's approval. Concord Hospital calls this The Concord Collaborative Care Model and reports "improved outcomes and high patient satisfaction."

Other hospitals are working to set up similar programs, but you don't have to sit idly by and wait for that to happen in your hospital. You can institute your own plan for "patient centered care" on the first day of hospitalization. That is the time to inform your admitting doctor, your nurses, and the attending physician that you expect to see and converse with the attending and the other members of the team *every* day at rounds. Your nurse can also notify the team of your wishes and should put a note on the front of your chart to alert the physicians that you insist on having a voice in your care. Don't let the meeting end before all your questions are answered. If a physician must leave, ask the person to commit to a return time when he or she won't be rushed. There is a very real power is having, and stating, expectations.

When the team enters your room, ask for their full attention and a detailed explanation of the plan for that day. What tests will be ordered? Are there any changes in medications? What treatment goals is the doctor hoping to reach today? What can you, the patient, do to assist in your care? Is the doctor aware of any glitches or problems from the day before, and how can you be sure they won't happen again today?

ATTENDING PHYSICIANS are the most senior doctors directly responsible for your care. Simply stated, they are the bosses of the house staff. Since they have completed their minimum three years of residency training and often have years of practical, hands-on experience, they are considered the more established physicians and can practice medicine unsupervised. (At the very least, every physician must complete medical school, pass national and state board examinations, and complete a three-year residency program before they can do this.)

Attending physicians not only provide medical care but are responsible for training the residents affiliated with the hospital. Ideally, they will review your admission notes, history, and physical exam findings within 24 hours of admission. At the very least, they should be co-signing consultations reports, operative reports, radiology reports, discharge summaries, and "Do Not Resuscitate" (DNR) orders. Ultimately, they are the ones who are responsible for the quality of care delivered to each patient under their watch. At large teaching hospitals, where there is an extensive hierarchy of physicians, they may also wear the hat of professor or researcher.

The attending physician might *orchestrate* your medical care, but she relies heavily on interns, residents or fellows to attend to the day-to-day details: writing orders, seeing patients, performing routine procedures. At one major medical center in San Francisco, the role was described to me as follows: "The attending physician should look at the chart everyday," but he "cannot be expected to do all the work" or be "physically present" for the large numbers of patients who have to be managed. Attending physicians should have the final say in important medical decisions, but this is not always the case.

The attending physician has a dual role then; she is a teacher and a caregiver. Consequently, she will spend as much or more time questioning residents and students than she will speaking to you. She may be so focused on the students, in fact, that she seems virtually unavailable to answer *your* questions. What this all means is that you cannot count on spending much time with her. Often the only contact the attending has with patients is during daily rounds. A group of doctors, led by the attending physician, quickly reviews the patient's progress and discusses plans for his care. Traditionally, rounds begin outside the patient's room in the hallway, and he is excluded from this critical strategic planning session. This is not quite as egregious a practice as it sounds. Doctors do need time to speak to each other without including you in every transaction. However, you are entitled to ask them to refocus their attention on you at some point. You do not have to be completely left out of the process. Once you have their attention, though, use it wisely. Ask important questions, not trivial ones, and think about how to phrase them ahead of time. This is not a social visit. It is a strategic planning session that sets the tone for the entire day and ensures that you are included every step of the way.

Since attending physicians are mentors to others, this is what you should expect from them as medical education leaders. They should lead by example. They ought to stand firm for full disclosure to a patient when a mistake has been made. They should include the patient in the medical process. They should be honest about their own fallibility and be willing to admit their mistakes. The goal of current patient safety experts is a "no blame" mentality, in which individuals don't have to assume personal responsibility for errors that can be attributed to a flaw in the "system." The rationale behind this is that hospital personnel will be more likely to admit their mistakes freely if they are not afraid of being blamed or disciplined. Errors are not supposed to be hidden because that makes it so much easier to repeat them. If, however, residents watch their supervisors sweep their mistakes under the rug, they are influenced to do the same. Why would one expect a first-year to raise his hand and admit to a faulty procedure when he has seen others lie and sail through the system without being censured? What incentive do young doctors have to reveal their oversights? In an article in the *New England Journal of Medicine,* a study was cited showing that "only 54 percent of House

Officers [house staff] had told their attending physician about the most serious errors they had committed in the previous year. Thirty-one percent of the errors reported in the study resulted in the patient's death." That is a staggering statistic, and the numbers will remain high unless an atmosphere of openness and honesty is fostered by the attending physicians. It is easy enough to hide serious situations with vague general statements that seem to account for complications and death. A death certificate might say that Mr. Jones died of "heart failure." That doesn't mean his heart was the only cause of his death. Perhaps the patient suffered through a post-operative infection or a surgical error, but these things may not be noted on death certificates. As the leader of his troop, the attending physician must put the truth about patient outcomes first.

Attendings should also treat patients with respect and dignity, thereby reinforcing the golden rule. They ought to stand as beacons for truthfulness, ethics and morality. I've stated what good healthcare leaders should do. Here's what they *should not* do: Lie by omission; mislead patients or their families in any way or ask other staff members to compromise their integrity by keeping silent about mistakes; blame patients, trainees, or other staff members when there is a mishap; shrug off their responsibility to search for ways of improving healthcare delivery, saying that "the system is too far gone to do anything about it." The attending is the one who sets the tone on the hospital floor. If he establishes an air of secrecy and blame, it fosters the practice of not admitting mistakes. This lays the groundwork for cover-up and for the continuation of mistakes that could be corrected.

FELLOWS operate at a level of responsibility just below attending physicians. They are physicians who have completed their residency in the recent past and have chosen to pursue a "fellowship," which is advanced training in a particular specialty. Their title, which is friendly and almost jovial, doesn't actually tell you a thing about what they do. In fact, the purpose of a fellowship is not to help the practitioner hone his bedside manner and be more sociable; it is to further his training in a specialized area of interest. A fellowship involves a variety of responsibilities including patient care, instruction of residents, participation in weekly conferences and varying amounts of research. But because of the demands of their research duties, fellows spend only a limited amount of time seeing patients. You are far more likely to encounter fellows at major medical centers that have ties to schools or research facilities.

What can you can expect from a fellow? She can order tests, may change your medication orders and request consultations by specialists. She may make a brief appearance in your room to introduce herself. "Hi. I'm Doctor Smith, and I will be checking on your progress." If this event doesn't occur, you may not even know that a fellow is helping to oversee your care. If you want to find out, you have to ask.

Fellows work closely with the attending physicians, who rely on them to assist in supervising residents by functioning as a back-up support when they are unavailable. A fellow who trains residents will review your record and has the authority to make decisions regarding your medical care, but you need to be aware that she is subordinate to the attending physician and even *her* treatment plans should be reviewed and approved by him. The fellow might not be visible to you, but she is important. Ask if a fellow is a member of your team and request a meeting with her in person. If this doctor is making life-and-death decisions about your body, you should make sure that you let her know how important it is to be kept informed about your care. You want to be sure she has looked over your medical history and is aware of any allergies or unusual conditions. Let her know if it is all right to speak to your friends or relatives about your medical issues so she won't be worried about breaching your confidentiality. In the event of a problem or complications, a fellow is yet another person to turn to for input, but don't expect a lot of hand-holding from this person because the reality is that helping to oversee your care is only a small part of her responsibility. Still, there is nothing unreasonable about expecting a face-to-face meeting with her soon after admission.

The next rung on the ladder is the complex RESIDENT classification. Upon graduation from medical school and satisfactory performance on state and national board exams, a student officially becomes an "MD," but he cannot work on his own, unsupervised. First, he has to complete a minimum of three years (a full 36 months) of hands-on training (residency). For you, the patient, this is a good thing. We don't want people flying solo whose only understanding of your body comes from a textbook. The human body is not like a washing machine; it is far too complex to be grasped by simply reading a user's manual. In the practice of medicine, one cannot overestimate the value of experience, hands-on training and intuition. Experience is especially important because there is a big difference between seeing something done a few times and assisting in a procedure dozens of times. With repetition comes added information and greatly increased skill levels. Often, experience is what leads a more seasoned doctor to act accurately and in a timely way on a hunch about a patient while the more inexperienced doctors run to a reference book to look up the symptoms.

For patients, the resident category can be the most perplexing and misleading in the whole medical hierarchy simply because, depending on the year of the resident, there are many levels of skill. A first-year resident who is on her first day on the job has literally just left the classroom. She has virtually no experience in diagnosing patients. And adding to the problem, titles can vary from institution to institution. For example, a new doctor can be called an intern in one hospital, a PGY1 (Post-graduate year 1) at another and an R1 (Resident year 1) at a third. So the patient has to remember the title as well as what the number after it corresponds to. The terms *intern, resident 1, 2, or 3, PGY 1, 2, or 3* may seem daunting at first, but gaining a basic understanding of their role and level of training is not a difficult task. These terms are important to your care, so don't brush them off by thinking it is too complicated or by assuming that they are all interchangeable.

You must know the level of experience of each physician entering your room long before a crisis occurs. In a crisis, people have to think quickly. If an emergency occurs, a nurse is probably the first person on the scene. It is the usual practice to start at the bottom and work her way up to the more experienced doctors. Technically, when she calls in a first-year resident, the nurse is meeting her obligation to inform a doctor of a change in a patient's status, but, of course, this person may not have the expertise to recognize the onset of a serious complication. By the time the less experienced resident decides that your symptoms warrant a look by someone more senior to him or her, it could be too late. If you or your advocate feel strongly that the situation is serious, you can immediately call for more senior personnel. In other words, you can jump a few notches in the chain and bypass the less experienced interns, thereby saving valuable time.

I wish I could state unequivocally that requesting an experienced doctor guarantees that the right decisions will be made about your care. As the following story shows, that is not always the case. Lewis Blackman's parents were smart enough to ask for an attending physician after a first-year resident four months out of school answered their original calls for help, but another resident arrived instead. Even though he was more experienced than the original responder, he lacked the intuition of a truly experienced doctor and missed obvious signs of life-threatening complications. Lewis was being operated on for a medical condition known as pectus excavatum: his breastbone sat too far within his chest cavity. To correct the condition, he had surgery: a metal bar was inserted in his chest to support the sunken breastbone. Three days after the operation, the boy complained of severe stomach pain. Later that day, Lewis's belly became bloated, his pulse increased, and he grew pale, sweaty and weak—all signs of shock. When the first-year resident, whom the nurse called in first, dismissed the signals and the parents didn't accept her diagnosis, an attending physician was requested. Lewis's parents assumed that the more confident physician who strode into the room was the attending physician, but he was actually the chief resident—in this case a 4th year general surgery resident just beginning his pediatric rotation. He essentially confirmed that it was nothing serious and told Lewis's mother that her son was constipated.

What Lewis had, in fact, was a serious condition. He was developing a perforated duodenal ulcer, which was a known complication of the pain medicine he was receiving. The ulcer had eaten a hole in his intestines and was causing infection and massive internal bleeding. Simple blood tests would have detected the infection, but they were not ordered. Instead, the 4th year surgery resident decided that Lewis should be treated with suppositories to treat his "constipation." The next morning when the nurse's aide was unable to detect a blood pressure reading (another sign of shock), a second-year resident tried several times to obtain another blood pressure reading and thought she got one that could be in the normal range. It was, however, a false reading; unknowingly, she recorded it in the chart and yet another chance to save this boy's life was lost. Within two hours, this healthy 15-year-old was dead. Dr. Gregg Korbon, an anesthesiologist and family friend, was later quoted in South Carolina's *The State* as saying, "Even a boy scout could have done better . . . it's hard to kill a healthy 15-year-old."

The tragedy of this case is that it exhibits a lethal combination of inattention to crucial details and a lack of experience. The chief resident seemed to take his cues from less experienced personnel and did not look deeply enough into the patient's situation. An attending physician would likely have recognized the severity of the problem and taken steps to prevent its continuance. If you or someone you love is undergoing a worsening in a condition, and you feel that a resident *of any level* is not up to the task, do not hesitate to call in an attending physician and *be sure that the person who arrives is indeed an attending physician.*

The ideal scenario during a hospital stay is to know the name of every doctor responsible for your care and his or her level of experience. This includes those who might be instructing or supervising your immediate physician. In a NEJM (*New England Journal of Medicine*) article, an anonymous resident said these chilling words: "I put in a central line today that was complicated by a pneumothorax [collapsed lung]. I had never done the procedure before, and I am not sure the resident who was supervising me had much more experience than I do." If the skill of the supervisor is barely higher than the one he is teaching, how confident can you be in the procedure? You certainly cannot count on staff to volunteer a statement like, "I'm not entirely sure of myself here, and the guy whose watching over me has only done this once, but don't worry; we'll figure it out." It's important to ascertain the experience level of everyone involved in decisions about your body.

Many people actually write down the names and ranks of the staff because they know how valuable it is, when asking for help, to be able to rattle off a specific title. For example, consider the difference between saying, "I think my child needs to be seen by someone else" and saying, "My son is having symptoms that alarm me, and I want him evaluated by the attending physician as soon as possible." If you just ask for "someone," you could get a first-year resident just out of medical school. The more specific you can be, the better the odds are that the person attending you will be up to the job. If you leave it to the system, the doctor with the least experience may be the one with the greatest responsibility for your care.

Lewis Blackman's family used some of their malpractice settlement to help enact the Lewis Blackman Hospital Patient Safety Act in South Carolina. Adopted in June, 2005, the act contains four basic, simple and potentially life-saving provisions. 1. All hospital personnel are required to wear name badges clearly stating their legal names and their job title. Students, interns and residents will be noted as such on their name badges. 2. Prior to or upon admission, patients will be provided written information identifying the role of the attending physician and resident physicians in their care. 3. The nursing staff is required to contact the attending physician at the patient's request. If the patient wants to call the attending themselves, the nurse will provide the number and assist in making the call. 4. Hospitals shall have a patient assistance program in place for patients to voice concerns and to be able to contact the hospital administration so they can assess a situation and respond appropriately. Patients in every state should expect and insist on these reasonable accommodations—ask that they be done and tell the administration at your hospital that you would like them to follow suit and voluntarily adopt the provisions of the Lewis Blackman Hospital Patient Safety Act.

It is important to understand that the more experienced residents are always trying to move on with their training and have less time for bedside care. First-year residents will not be assisting much in the operating room, delivering a set of premature twins, or supervising the progress of residents beneath them. Instead, they are more likely to be the ones evaluating why Mr. Smith hasn't urinated in several hours, which is no trivial matter if Mr. Smith is teetering on the brink of shock.

Intern, Resident-1 or PGY-1 — (The term *intern* usually only refers to first-year residents.) In August 1999, Marlene Joseph went into labor at Albert Einstein Hospital in the Bronx. A first-year resident asked the woman's husband to step outside, and he assumed that she was simply going to prep his wife for surgery, but when he left the room, she actually began an epidural procedure, a skill she was not proficient in. She ended up aiming the catheter in the wrong direction and hitting the spinal cord, thereby introducing air into the patient's bloodstream. Mrs. Joseph's health declined rapidly as the air bubble lodged in an area that stopped her breathing. She had to be kept alive using a manual ventilation bag, and her daughter had to be delivered via an emergency C-section. Upon seeing what she had done, the resident tried to cover up the disastrous procedure by taking out the catheter and saying that the patient had begun to code before she had ever begun the epidural. After Mrs. Joseph died and an autopsy was performed, naturally the truth came out. What this story shows is two things: one, what can happen when an resident acts without proper supervision on a procedure she isn't trained to do, and two, how easily an inexperienced first-year doctor can panic and try to cover up a mistake.

First-year residents are easy to recognize. They are the new kids on the block and are, understandably, nervous. They spend a lot of time flipping through small notebooks of condensed medical facts, and their beside manner is, at best, unrefined. It is not uncommon to see them walking around talking to themselves and triple-checking their calculations because they don't have the experience to be completely confident in their decisions. They seem to obsess over minute details. They have to confirm their opinions and decisions with someone else and then justify their rationale. In addition, they must be sure to impress second and third- year residents, attending physicians, fellows, and staff physicians. They are constantly being scrutinized and evaluated, and their place in the residency program is contingent on performance. This is the nature of the game, so don't expect first-year residents to have the same skills or to perform at the same level as an experienced doctor.

One day these first-years are in an insulated classroom environment safely removed from the complexities of the human body, and the next day they are in an emergency room splattered with blood. They are expected to make serious decisions that the patient has to live with–or die with. A tragic example is Dr. Karl Shipman, who had surgery to set a broken wrist, but shortly after being released from the hospital, his body was wracked with pain. He was eventually admitted to the ICU of the Denver hospital that he, himself, happened to work at. Unfortunately for Dr. Shipman, the person in charge that night was an intern just out of medical school who did not recognize that her patient had a staph infection raging through his system. In a case where infection is suspected, it is standard to order blood cultures and to start antibiotic therapy after the cultures are obtained. Instead, potentially life-saving antibiotics weren't administered soon enough and Dr. Shipman's liver and kidneys began to fail. An intensivist (ICU specialist) was available in the hospital but was not brought in to consult in time to make a difference. In all likelihood, an experienced intensive care doctor would have recognized the serious nature of Dr. Shipman's situation. Tragically, before antibiotics and other interventions had a chance to take effect, Dr. Shipman went into complete cardiovascular collapse including shock and respiratory failure, which are common complications of sepsis. He died from the infection.

In addition to dealing with the enormity of their responsibility, first-years are exhausted and sleep deprived; nevertheless, they still have to think on their feet and be accurate. As was true in Dr. Shipman's case, this could be the person whose choices decide whether you live or die. The unrelenting fatigue, stress, and chaos experienced by new doctors all takes a physical, mental and emotional toll. And weighing over them is the fact that they have now reached the status where they can even be named in a lawsuit against the hospital. You will find that they tend to rely heavily on nurses, who have much more hands-on experience than they do, for procedural guidance. This is actually beneficial to patients since the more experienced nurses can offer suggestions or catch possible errors before they are made.

Not only do first- year residents work long hours under enormous amounts of stress, but they may be on call more nights per month than the more experienced second and third- year residents. Ridiculously long hours have been a part of the medical education process since its inception, and first-year residents may clearly be in a groggy state, apparent even to their patients. On a national level, residents may work as many as 80 hours a week and often go as long as 36 hours without sleep. It is amazing that we continue to accept these dangerously long shifts, with the inherent risks to patient safety that they pose, as an integral part of medical training.

To their credit, though, first-year residents seem well aware of their lack of experience and do not regard the fact that they may need more guidance as a personal or professional failure. As an example, in 1998, the residents at a major San Francisco medical center negotiated to postpone their pediatric oncology rotation until the second year of their residency. A resident I spoke to stated that they simply weren't confident that they were ready to handle the complexities of medical oncology case management. After their complaints, the pediatric oncology rotation became part of the second-year curriculum, not the first year. We should applaud these beginners who recognized their limitations and were not willing to put their own careers ahead of public safety.

Resident-2 or PGY-2 (Post-graduate year two) refers to the second year of residency training. The R-2s or PGY-2s assume more responsibility. They will work with patients, but also operate in a teaching capacity for first-year residents, helping to train and supervise them. Every time they go up a level in the residency program, it means that their experience, confidence and ability have increased also. Somehow, the improvement always seemed most obvious to me when interns were jumping from the R-1 to R-2 phase. As hard as first year is, at least these residents are not put in the position of having to supervise other people, (although they may occasionally have medical students, whose duties are extremely limited, tagging along behind them).

For patients, having a second-year attend to them is a double-edged sword. They might be getting a doctor who is more experienced, but that person also has the added burden of supervising others after only one year of training. That prospect would be daunting to anyone. You, the patient, aren't in a position to change hospital policy on staffing, but that doesn't mean you're helpless. You can rely on your initial impressions of the treating physician to determine if he is competent, inquire about his experience level, and insist on being seen by a more senior physician if you have doubts about the ability of a resident to manage your case.

Medicine continues to let novices take on the role of supervisor, even though they're still at the lower end of the learning curve, and even though this practice has been linked to a number of serious medical errors. Did you know that you could be wheeled into an emergency room in the middle of the night, and the physician in charge of your care could only be in the first week of her second-year residency training? That is practically the same as having a PGY1 left to find out why your breathing passage is obstructed or why your heart is palpating wildly. Some emergencies involve a broken thumb, but others are life and death episodes. If this inexperienced doctor has to tend to your emergency, plus be on call to supervise underlings, how much expert attention can they be expected to provide on a consistent basis?

You must remind yourself that if you feel your safety is being compromised, you can always summon more senior doctors from another part of the hospital to consult or assist. Residents may resist paging senior staff because they are always being evaluated on their ability to be self-reliant and handle emergencies on their own. These are the benchmarks of their ability during medical training. If the PGY2 is constantly paging the attending physician because the nurses, patients, or their families are expressing doubts about her performance, this could quickly become an embarrassing liability for her. As sorry as you may be about the impact on her career, it is not your concern. Your concern is your health. If you have persistent doubts about the second-year's capacities, call in a more senior doctor and be specific in your wording. Say, "I feel my situation warrants being seen by the attending physician, and I am asking that you contact him. I have asked my nurse to document in my chart that I've made this request." Or, "I am requesting a consultation by a specialist or qualified surgeon for the severe pain in my stomach." If the resident resists, tell her you are aware that she always has the option to consult with more senior staff members and you are insisting, politely, that she do so.

Resident-3 or PGY-3 — Again, the third-year is considerably more experienced and assured than the second-year students. While the third-year medical residents are confident and knowledgeable, what is gained in experience tends to be offset by their somewhat hardened persona and an intense focus on their future. They are about to go forth and earn a living, and they know it. They are often preoccupied by questions of where they will practice, what medical group they will join, whether they ought to get more training, and so on. From the first day of any residency program, a physician's sights are set on this finish line. Perhaps it cannot be any other way if they are to survive the grueling gauntlet of medical education. They have studied

for years, made countless personal sacrifices, and paid a heavy emotional and financial price for this one goal. They've seen a lot of suffering and death and have had to develop a tempered detachment.
Unfortunately, this can make them less empathic to their patients
and less fascinated by their patients' medical problems.

Since attending physicians and fellows are focused on teaching
residents and on overall patient management and the residents are
focused on completing their program successfully and impressing
their superiors, it is easy to see why the focus rarely seems to be on
the patient as an individual. This was explained to me by a patient
relations staff member at a major San Francisco medical center as
"the teaching hospital trade-off." The patient has the advantage of a
high-tech team approach, the newest procedures available, and the
opinion of specialists. On the other hand, the medical environment
can be chaotic and impersonal, and the individual patient can fall
between the cracks. As the patient, you just don't want the trade-off
to result in a setback in your recovery just so a resident can gain new
experience.

Resident-4 or PGY-4 — Some programs offer a fourth-year elective position for further training in a specific area or for the opportunity to
serve as chief resident, but a fourth year of residency is usually not a
requirement of a residency program. Certain residents will, at this
point, seek a fellowship to gain experience in clinical areas, research,
or to explore potential faculty positions.

Fifth and Sixth Year Residents are usually training to become surgeons.
Hence, they spend additional years learning the art of surgery.

Chief Residents are a select group. They are third-years who have
either been elected by fellow residents or appointed by the program
director to occupy a unique position of increased responsibility and
accountability. The duties of a chief resident fall into four major
categories: administrative—scheduling on-call duties, rotations and
vacations; clinical—seeing patients after they have been admitted and

had their medical history taken by the residents; academic—arranging for lectures, guest speakers, and conferences for the residency program; supervisory—managing the residents, delegating duties, and evaluating resident proficiency.

The fact that the chief resident has so many demanding duties means that the chosen individual must clearly have demonstrated leadership ability and shown composure under pressure. This person is the official liaison between the faculty and the residents. If residents have a problem with a staff member or a hospital policy, he is their first sounding board. Yet he is not only a voice for residents; he must also be a voice for the system. As one who works in a gray zone between the two, he must move effortlessly back and forth between them dozens of times a day.

In addition to the above duties, the chief medical resident is often responsible for ensuring that the Emergency Department is adequately staffed with residents at all times. (Some people think this is a job in and of itself.) He may also have other duties such as managing the monthly Morbidity and Mortality Conference, the arena where doctors are supposed to admit their mistakes to each other and evaluate why certain treatment plans were unsuccessful.

An attending physician may actually prove to be more accessible than the chief resident, simply because the chief resident has so many responsibilities. Consequently, if you find yourself in a position that warrants a more senior doctor, you might be better off asking for an attending physician rather then the "chief." The attending may be more familiar with your case and reach your bedside sooner.

HOSPITALISTS — Recently, a new group of physicians have risen in prominence in the American healthcare system; they are known as hospitalists. These people focus a great deal of their medical practice on the sole care of hospitalized patients. Some hospitalists only work in hospitals and have no private practice of their own, while others may continue their private practice on a limited basis but devote most of their time to working with hospitalized patients.

There are advantages to using hospitalists. Since they work on-site, they are more available, and since they practice inside hospital walls more often, they probably have more expertise in meeting the needs of hospitalized patients. In addition, they have greater familiarity with hospital rules and procedures (and the potential for cost savings resulting from more streamlined, coordinated care) than a private physician. The medical community has been divided on their use, however. Some are concerned that the hospital skills of primary care physicians in private practice will atrophy from lack of use. Some also have their doubts about physician and patient acceptance and the possible erosion of established doctor/patient relationships because the hospitalist's patient pool is largely made up of people who are complete strangers to them; they have no ongoing interpersonal relationships with them.

In spite of this, a hospitalist could be an asset to you, the patient. This in-house physician who specializes in micro-managing your care may be more efficient at reviewing the copious amounts of continuously updated information, reviewing test results, and planning treatment, especially if this is what he does all day, every day. In theory, he would know exactly whom to call and what hoops to jump through to send you home healthy with the optimum of efficiency. He can function as a stable, constant and accessible coordinator of medical care.

Yet there are potential drawbacks to consider. Things can certainly get dicey if a hospitalist feels that his loyalty belongs primarily to his employer and not to his patients. Of course, hospitals are only going to hire hospitalist's who subscribe to the philosophy and the politics of the institution. It is highly unlikely that a hospitalist who wants to "buck the system" in any way will keep his job. If you are aware that your hospital employs a hospitalist who is in charge of your care, you will want to be realistic about his motivation. Of course, his loyalty could be divided between you and the entity who signs his paychecks. In other words, be prepared to stand up to him or her if your care seems lacking in any way.

MEDICAL STUDENTS — There is another group of individuals who are not yet medical doctors who may be part of the team managing your care—students. Those in the third and fourth year of classroom work do clerkships or rotations, which allow them to work in the residency program so they can gain hands-on experience working with patients, albeit experience of a limited nature. The rotations last for a set period of time and involve a realistic number of hours since medical students still spend most of their time in the classroom. These students will take medical histories, assess vital signs, and even, remarkably, may be able to write orders in your chart. The general policy is that these orders must be checked and signed by a MD, but given the busyness of a hospital setting, oversights can occur. The greater risk for patients is that orders written by a student may not be reviewed in a timely manner, or they may be implemented by nurses or other staff members who don't realize that the author was a student.

If students are part of your medical team, ask if they will be writing orders in your chart. You will know they're medical students by their identification badges. You must make a point of scrutinizing all hospital badges, and if you are unable to see clearly, you must ask what is printed on them. By no means should you assume that all the people wearing scrubs or stethoscopes around their neck are bona fide doctors. The next question to ask is who will review and sign these orders and at what intervals. When encountering students, ask them to sign their name clearly with the designation "medical student" printed underneath—a clear signal that this recommendation must be double-checked (this also applies for nursing students). Also find out the name of the physician who is ultimately responsible for decisions about your care and inquire how she can be reached in case of questions or confusion. You will want to ask your nurse to be extra vigilant in assuring that any orders or notes written by medical and nursing students are reviewed and signed by licensed physicians and registered nurses.

REGISTERED NURSES comprise the largest segment of healthcare workers, and because they're the most hands-on of all hospital caregivers, they often function as the most powerful advocates for patients. Registered nurses must attend a state-approved school of nursing and may obtain a two-year associate degree (ADN), a diploma based on a three-year hospital program (ASN) or a baccalaureate degree in nursing (BSN) after the completion of a four-year university program. Registered nurses must maintain a valid and current license or certificate of registration and are bound by the guidelines of the Nursing Practice Act. In many states, a prerequisite for license renewal for RN's is the completion of dozens of hours of continuing education requirements.

Unlike most other hospital staff, nurses spend a great majority of their time providing direct patient care, and they are often the eyes and ears for busy physicians. They work at the patient's bedside, which places them right at the center of the action, a position from which they are the most likely to notice subtle changes in a patient's status. Nurses are also responsible for educating patients (and their families) about the nature of the illness and the recovery. Consequently, they are usually the ones who are dealing with their patient's concerns and fears, with family members, and with home care issues. The nurses are the practitioners who know the tried-and-true anecdotal remedies that offer solutions for those seemingly minor but intensely annoying conditions. In other words, their advice can significantly increase a patient's quality of life.

Nurses may not be at the very top of the medical hierarchy, but they have possibly the most complex responsibilities. They are continuously caught in the middle of a huge, unwieldy bureaucracy. They are often underpaid and overworked with demands being made on them on an hourly basis by people who are sick, fearful, in pain and possibly even dying. In spite of the constant pressure, though, nurses cannot let their frustrations interfere with their duties. Employees in other industries frequently have time to sit around at the water fountain and complain or meet in the coffee room for a gripe session to let off steam. Nurses have no such luxury. They are far too busy.

Nurses interact with a daunting array of people including doctors, pharmacists, lab personnel, social workers, clergy, housekeeping staff and assistive personnel. They probably have the most complete view of the healthcare system as a whole. It could be argued that everything ultimately revolves around them and around what transpires right at the patient's bedside. They see all the components of the healthcare pie and observe, on a daily basis, the politics that decide who gets what share of the resources. Financial entities, physician medical groups, hospital administrations, insurance companies, and patients and their loved ones are all vying for a larger share of healthcare expenditures. Nurses are the healthcare provider group most free from outside influences and political and financial incentives. This means that their motivation remains pure: they simply want to see their patients cared for in a safe, well-managed environment and to be compensated fairly for their services.

A decade of research supports one important assertion: a greater ratio of RNs to patients in a hospital results in a significant decrease in complications and mortality for patients. This makes even more sense when you consider the complex patient assessment duties that nurses perform. Contrary to popular belief, nurses don't just take your blood pressure and record a value in your chart. They actually interpret the significance of the numbers when applied to your overall clinical picture. Because of this, nurses are often the staff members who detect the first signs of a complication. When a nurse does notice a potential problem and alerts your doctor at the earliest juncture, he or she has just dramatically increased your chances of leaving the hospital alive.

Just as it is with the other healthcare practitioners, it is critical to look at nametags and to understand what various classifications mean within the nursing staff.

NURSING SUPERVISORS include both charge nurses and nurse managers.

Charge Nurses are responsible for all the nursing care in a ward or unit during each assigned shift. They perform the daily supervision and management of the unit and function as the immediate supervisor for the bedside nurses. The charge nurse is the logical "go-to" person for nurses who encounter any difficulties during their shift and the first person to contact if there is a problem with your nurse that cannot be resolved quickly and amicably.

Nurse Managers are part of the leadership team and are considered "nursing executives." Nurse Managers may be required to have a master's degree and practical experience. They have duties such as recruiting and retaining staff, planning both short-term and long-term staffing needs, ensuring compliance with regulatory standards, evaluating the performance of staff and having input on both promotions and terminations, working on continuity of care issues and cost-containment strategies. Nurse Managers may be on-call 24 hours a day and are the direct supervisors of Charge Nurses.

ADVANCED PRACTICE NURSES are registered nurses who have completed advanced training beyond the basic criteria that all RNs must fulfill. They meet higher educational and clinical requirements than other nursing groups. Within this category, there are two groups: nurse practitioners (NP) and clinical nurse specialists (CNS). Both have masters or doctorate degrees in nursing, allowing them to assume greater responsibility in patient care, teaching, case management, and consulting.

Nurse Practitioners work closely with physicians and are qualified to diagnose and treat common illnesses and injuries. A NP can actually function as a patient's main healthcare provider, meaning that this is the person you would go to with a sore throat or a persistent ache. To some degree, NPs can function as internists. They tend to have more personal contact with clients because they spend more time talking with them than physicians do. More and more patients are happy to rely on them as the "go to" person for their medical care. Nurse practitioners will assess what might be wrong with the patient and then direct him onto the next step. A majority of states even allow them to write prescriptions. NPs are growing in number because they represent a cost-saving feature for the hospital, and patients seem to like the personal attention.

The duties NPs perform are far-reaching and clearly go beyond the level of care delivered by a registered nurse. They may take medical histories and perform annual physical exams; diagnose and treat acute illnesses, infections, and injuries; diagnose and manage chronic conditions such as diabetes, heart disease, or high blood pressure; order diagnostic tests such as blood work, X-rays, or EKGs; and prescribe medications (when allowed by individual state law). They may also order physical or occupational therapy, well childcare, and immunizations.

The nurse practitioner's far-reaching goals are to provide individualized care, to prevent disease, and to increase patient education. They inform and educate patients about healthcare issues and encourage them to become active participants (i.e., empowered patients) in their quest for wellness. They are often looked to as a model for high-quality healthcare that is also cost effective.

A Clinical Nurse Specialist functions as an expert whose focus is on some specific area of nursing practice. For example, a CNS may specialize in treating surgical, diabetic, geriatric, cardiovascular, psychiatric or pediatric patients. Treating a certain group of patient's day in and day out gives these nurses superior skills in assessing an individual's clinical picture. Typically, a CNS can be expected to divide her time among several areas: seeing patients; teaching patients, families and other nurses; conducting research projects; providing consultations for patients and coordinating necessary consultations from other healthcare professionals; and managing cases.

The management skills of Clinical Nurse Specialists allow them to function as highly effective medical treatment managers who organize and oversee resources and services, work to ensure the continuity of care, and implement new improvements and standards for healthcare delivery in their institutions. For all practical purposes, advanced practice nurses indirectly help reduce the unnecessary healthcare expenditures that often result from ineffective or uncoordinated care.

LICENSED PRACTICAL NURSE (LPN) OR LICENSED VOCATIONAL NURSE (LVN)

are simply different terms for the same practitioner. They are not RNs, but they do provide basic nursing services under the direction and supervision of a physician or a registered nurse. LVNs must successfully complete a course of approximately 1,500 hours, or one year, of instruction. They are licensed by the state in which they work. LVNs will perform duties such as taking vital signs, monitoring venous catheters, writing notes in the patient's chart, administering medications as ordered by a physician and communicating information about a patient's status to registered nurses. With additional certification, LVNs may be able to draw blood or administer IV medications.

Each state has its own Nursing Practice Act, or some kind of guideline, that attempts to determine the scope of practice for practical nurses. This said, there is still ongoing discussion and debate (and there have even been lawsuits) concerning the level of nursing care that LVNs should be allowed deliver and whether their duties should be expanded. States vary in what they will allow LVNs to do and in the degree of direct supervision they need. Unfortunately, the guidelines are often generalized and in some cases ambiguous. Many people are concerned that this situation sets the stage for LVNs to be assigned responsibilities that go beyond their level of training and expertise just to contain costs or to solve the nursing shortage crisis. LVN salaries are lower than those of RNs'; substituting LVNs for RNs has become a common cost-cutting practice in hospitals across the nation.

In general, LVNs perform basic assessments on patients, which allow them to collect data. The simplest types of duties are taking a blood pressure or temperature reading and recording it in a patient's chart. If a value is out of the normal range, the LVN should be able to recognize it and notify a registered nurse or physician. She should not come to her own conclusions as to the significance of the value or the need for a change in the course of action. LVNs are not supposed to interpret or evaluate data, since this requires the complex knowledge and the application of the clinical judgment skills of a RN. In other words, LVN's obtain and report pieces of the information puzzle, but they do not diagnose, make referrals, or alter the patient's treatment plan based on their findings.

It is important for patients to know that it is not appropriate for a RN to merely "signoff" on the data collected by a LVN. Registered nurses must personally observe and evaluate the patients under their care. They are the ones who are legally responsible for the nursing care that is being provided.

UNLICENSED ASSISTIVE PERSONNEL (UAP) are unlicensed individuals who work in an assistive role to a licensed nurse. Ideally, UAPs help patients with their *basic* human needs including feeding, drinking, walking, positioning, grooming, toileting, dressing, etc. Increasingly, licensed nurses are being put in the position of delegating more complex nursing duties to assistive personnel because their institutions are hiring fewer registered nurses. The trend in hospitals to reduce the number of higher paid registered nurses and hire additional lesser-paid UAPs is very disturbing, and it is not good news for patients. These workers include Nurses Aides (NA), Nursing Assistants and Patient Care Assistants (PCA). The exact titles vary, but you will know by looking at their nametags that they are not an RN or LVN.

The training requirements for these workers vary widely from state to state. While doing research for this book, I found programs for a PCA that were as short as 80 hours. The minimum age and education requirements for a PCA in some states are being merely 16 to18 years old and having a high school diploma. Some of these unlicensed workers have less than 40 hours of hands-on hospital training when they graduate from the program. Many UAPs do successfully complete a state exam for certification, but in many states it is not required for employment.

The list of potential duties UAPs can perform is often frighteningly vague and may be too challenging for their skill level and knowledge. Such duties may include asepsis (preventing infections), changing dressings, catheterizing, inserting feeding tubes, assessing vital signs, imparting nutrition principles, providing post-op care, recognizing emergency situations, communicating information to patients, and having legal and ethical responsibilities. This is an amazingly daunting list for workers with so little training. Clearly, it can lead to an increased risk of complications for patients.

Here is one tragic example. In a skilled nursing facility, a newly hired nursing assistant was assigned to "feed" a patient who was unable to swallow, and thus had a feeding tube in his throat. The nurse naturally assumed that the assistant understood that a patient who cannot swallow should not be fed solid food. She was wrong. The assistant bypassed the tube and tried putting food in his mouth. The patient ended up dying after choking on eggs and toast that he was never supposed to be given. In 1994, *Time Magazine* reported the death of Rebecca Strunk, a 46-year-old patient who went in for a hysterectomy and came out with a lacerated bowel. Astonishingly, the individuals who were making important judgments about Mrs. Strunk's care were actually "patient care technicians," this hospital's term for a UAP. They made a diagnosis and charted her discomfort as routine "incisional pain." By the time her fever and other symptoms were obvious to everybody, she was reaching a critical point. The technician who noted the symptoms in the chart was never supposed to assess what they meant or how serious they were. That wasn't her job. And the nurses and residents never noticed the observations and said, "Wait a minute. That person isn't qualified to make a judgment call on the cause of a patient's pain. We'd better investigate." In the end, the hospital paid $3 million for a wrongful death settlement. It would have been cheaper and much more ethical to pay trained personnel to assess patient's symptoms rather than assigning the task to an unqualified technician.

My intention here is not to undermine assistive personnel. They do play a vital role in the hospital setting. My only point is that their responsibilities ought to be commensurate with their training. Originally, they were hired to relieve registered nurses of simple, yet time-consuming, tasks. In theory, this arrangement was supposed to give the highly trained RN more time for important patient care duties such as dispensing medications on time and consulting with physicians. But what started as an adjunctive position to relieve highly trained nurses of simple tasks has, for many hospitals, segued into a cost-cutting solution. Some hospitals are content with having a very limited number of registered nurses on staff and relying on UAPs to perform increasingly difficult functions that were traditionally assigned to RNs or LVNs. As a patient, you need to be aware of this trend. Look for signs that lesser-trained individuals are caring for you by reading name tags. If you feel that your safety is being compromised in any way, do not hesitate to speak up. You do not want to contract a staph infection, choke on a piece of beef, or be wheeled in for an invasive exam you don't need, just because an 18-year-old trained for only a number of weeks doesn't fully comprehend their duties.

A real crisis in our healthcare system is occurring right now. Registered nurses are responsible for more patients than ever before, and the patient population is often more seriously ill. Consequently, nurses have less time than ever to evaluate the status of their patients, to educate and comfort patients or their family members, to communicate with physicians and other allied healthcare professionals, and to document information in the record. In addition, nurses are supposed to supervise UAPs and assess their skill levels. They weren't really trained to assess which assistants can take instruction and run with it and which ones have to have their hand held all the time. Because the job descriptions of UAPs are constantly expanding and can vary from hospital to hospital, it places an additional burden on the RN to know which tasks are appropriate or even legal, to delegate to them. A recent nursing school graduate I interviewed for this book confirmed that she had received "one, maybe two, hours" of instruction regarding the delegation of duties to assistive personnel. Just because a certificate states that a person is able to work in a hospital or nursing home as an aide does not mean that he or she will have the same level of comprehension, ability or competence as another will. Duties and assignments need to reflect this reality.

Ideally, a patient who knows in advance that she will be checking into a hospital can telephone the hospital administrator or patient relations department and inquire about this issue. State that you would prefer to have a registered nurse actually tending to you, not just supervising your care from a distance. Ask for the hospital's policy on UAPs and what duties they are allowed to perform. Be clear that you want the more highly trained RNs dispensing your medications, inserting catheters and changing dressings. The hospital may not guarantee that your wishes will be fulfilled, but it will be acutely aware that you are an informed, motivated patient. If it receives a number of inquiries like yours, it might be prompted to consider adjusting its hiring practices in order to satisfy an ever more educated and demanding public. Even if you are hospitalized unexpectedly, you or a loved one can always phone the administrator or public relations department right from your room. You can also speak to the charge nurse or the director of nursing about your expectations to assure that you receive the highest quality nursing care available.

The American medical system is not malevolent, but it can be careless. For instance, several years ago Indiana Attorney General Pamela Carter discovered that housekeeping and janitorial staff members were actually providing patient care services in several hospitals in her state. Housekeeping staff who were assigned to clean rooms were occasionally asked to dispense medications. In this case, government stepped in and put an end to the problem before anyone was hurt. Sometimes, though, it is up to patients to stand up for their own rights.

Action Steps

- Know that you can *always* be seen by a more experienced physician. Ask specifically for the Attending Physician if you have serious questions about the decisions made by residents.

- Inquire if the person who enters your room is indeed the Attending Physician. If someone else was sent in their place, be sure that you make it completely clear that you are still waiting for and expecting the Attending Physician to consult on your case.

- If you are denied access to the attending physician, *and you feel that you or a loved one is being placed in jeopardy,* write a note explaining that you requested, but did not see, the attending physician. Ask for your narrative to be added to your medical record. Sign, date and ask for a copy to keep.

- Realize that the House Staff can alter orders that you thought were firm. Be sure that you stay up-to-date on the most recent plan for your care. Ask to be notified if there are any changes.

- Have an advocate at the hospital to be able to speak with the doctors at "rounds," if you are unable to do this for yourself. Ask the medical staff to use the Concord Hospital model and include you and/or your advocate during rounds.

- Ask if your nurse is an R.N. and ask that a registered nurse perform such duties as dispensing medication, starting IV's and monitoring your vital signs. Only R.N.'s are trained to critically evaluate and make decisions about your need for additional care based on the numbers obtained from vital signs and the observations notes in your chart.

- Remember that staffing may be low on weekends or during holiday times. Try to schedule elective procedures other times.

- Always have a means to contact your surgeon in case of an emergency. When we were scheduling my teenage son for knee surgery, one of the first questions I asked each surgeon we saw for a consultation if he or she would be staying in town the first few days after the procedure and if he or she could provide me with a direct number to be used only in the case of an emergency. I would not have been comfortable any other way and the doctors were all very supportive and accommodating. You can be sure that they would want the same access to the surgeon if their own child was being operated on.

- Ask if your hospital utilizes Rapid Response Teams. A RRT is a group of highly-trained hospital staff members who respond to a sudden decline in a patient's health. If your loved one is deteriorating quickly, ask that the Rapid Response Team be called.

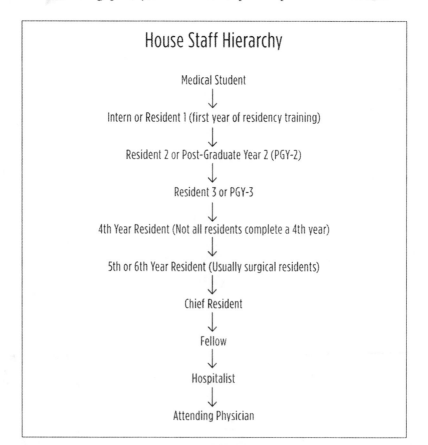

House Staff Hierarchy

Medical Student
↓
Intern or Resident 1 (first year of residency training)
↓
Resident 2 or Post-Graduate Year 2 (PGY-2)
↓
Resident 3 or PGY-3
↓
4th Year Resident (Not all residents complete a 4th year)
↓
5th or 6th Year Resident (Usually surgical residents)
↓
Chief Resident
↓
Fellow
↓
Hospitalist
↓
Attending Physician

Chapter Three

Infection Control and Prevention

How to Fight Infection in the Hospital and at Home

"Two million patients develop a hospital-acquired infection in the United States each year. Of that number, 90,000 die as a result of those infections."

– Dr. William Jarvis of the Centers for Disease Control

nfections that occur as a result of hospitalization are called *nosocomial infections*. The Center for Disease Control defines them as infections that arise a minimum of 48 hours after hospitalization; this length of time presumably excludes infections that were developing prior to admission. The CDC might monitor nosocomial infection rates but it does not require every healthcare institution to disclose numbers regarding its own infection rates. Since there is no federal mandate requiring all hospitals to report infection rates, the public's ability to learn about hospital infections is dependent upon vigilant monitoring by the institutions themselves and by complete honesty on their part in reporting problems. Decades of relying primarily on the honor system has not resulted in the disclosure of every event, and we still do not have all the raw data we need to ward off a virtual epidemic of completely preventable infections.

The price we pay for nosocomial infections is staggering. In 1995, it was estimated that they cost our healthcare system 4.5 billion dollars a year and the loss of one life every six minutes! A 2001 study in the journal *Emerging Infectious Diseases* estimated a 2.5 to 10 percent rate of hospital-acquired infections with a mortality rate of 875,000 to 3.5 million. Because our healthcare system has managed costs so effectively, these days only the sickest patients—hence, the most susceptible to infection—get admitted to hospitals. So many hospitals are now nothing more than giant intensive care units. Aggressive strategies that cut costs for institutions, but reduce the infection control budget for patients, have inevitably contributed to increased infection rates.

Hospitals today also find themselves with a lot of older patients. The combination of the aged and those who need more advanced and more invasive medical care (especially in the areas of transplantation and cancer therapy) has left hospitals with a significantly more immune-compromised patient population. Nosocomial infections are more likely to occur in patients whose immune systems are not functioning at optimum levels because of age, illness, or previous medical or surgical treatments. As one would expect, the highest rates are found in pediatric and adult intensive care units (ICUs), where hospital-acquired infections are approximately three times higher than in other areas of the hospital. A majority of these infections occur in particular areas of the body: surgical incisions, the urinary tract, and in the bloodstream. But patients in ICUs often require surgery, urinary catheters, and multiple invasive catheters in their veins (intravenous lines-IVs), so of course the staff is constantly invading physical environments known for their susceptibility to infection.

Ostensibly, we expect hospitals to have higher numbers of bacteria and greater varieties of pathogens than other places. And while it is also to be expected that big hospitals will care for larger numbers of critically ill patients, meaning they may always have higher infection percentages, they should not be allowed to use this as an excuse for rampant infection rates. Instead, there should be a call to action for more vigilant and carefully monitored infection control measures.

In 2000, the Institute of Medicine reported that hospital infections result in at least 90,000 deaths a year. A series in July of 2002 by reporter Michael Berens of the *Chicago Tribune* titled "Unhealthy Hospitals" puts the figure at 107,000 patient deaths a year, with as many as 75 percent of the them preventable. This number surpasses every other cause of accidental death in the United States and represents a serious ongoing threat to public health. Unlike other medical issues that create intense media coverage and heightened public awareness, this threat has long remained a dangerous secret. But this is a mistake because keeping the public in the dark about infection statistics has excluded a powerful ally: the patients themselves.

Can patients or their family members really reverse the odds of acquiring a nosocomial infection? The answer to that question is a resounding yes, since so many of them are *totally preventable*. If your risk for infection is greater than normal, a detailed medical history, a physical exam, and the proper blood studies should give your physician enough information to let you know the extra lengths you must go to protect yourself. But for patients *at all risk levels*, there are simple, specific strategies they can utilize during their hospital stay to reduce their chances of developing an infection.

Basic Precautions

"Basic precautions" (which may also be referred to as standard precautions or universal precautions) is a term used to define the fundamental actions required to prevent the transmission of disease between healthcare workers and their patients. These "barrier" type precautions were established by the CDC and were designed to limit a healthcare worker's exposure to contaminated blood and bodily fluids. An added benefit is that these precautions also work in reverse—they protect patients from exposure to pathogens being transported by their caregivers.

Universal precautions are to be used by healthcare workers for all patients, whether or not they have any signs of an infectious disease, and include regular hand cleansing, the appropriate use of gloves, and the use of masks, gowns, and protective eyewear when indicated. The fact that these safety measures may not be used religiously by healthcare workers represents a serious, ongoing threat to patient safety. A truly informed public would insist, in no uncertain terms, on compliance, and this would be the genesis of immediate reform.

Hand Hygiene

> *"Clean hands are the single most important factor in preventing the spread of dangerous germs and antibiotic resistance in healthcare settings."*
>
> – Julie Gerberding, MD, director of the CDC

Hand washing is a vital first-line defense against hospital-acquired infections, and studies done decades ago established a direct correlation between hand washing and significant reductions in infection rates. The CDC reports that thorough hand washing could save as many as 20,000 lives a year. A careful washing of the hands consumes only seconds of a healthcare worker's time and costs literally pennies to the institution. And the costs of *not* doing it are huge: the expense of hospital-acquired infections is now reaching into the billions of dollars; the loss of human life is incalculable. Consequently, a practice of stringently enforcing hand-washing rules would appear to be a no-brainer.

Unfortunately, in the healthcare system, convincing healthcare workers to practice the simple, basic act of hand washing has been an uphill battle. If you are a patient, all you have to do is observe the daily routine of those who take care of you to know that this "Holy Grail" of infection control is difficult to attain.

Respected medical journals have published articles reporting the dismal results of observational studies of hand washing compliance among healthcare workers. In November 1998, an *Infection Control and Hospital Epidemiology* article reported that the prevalence of hand washing at a teaching hospital in Ohio was a mere 30.2 percent. And this number remained stable for all three shifts: days, evenings and nights. The medical residents washed their hands 59.2 percent of the time, making them the most cooperative of all. The rest were compliant in descending order: Attending physicians washed their hands 37.4 percent of the time, followed by nurses at 32.6 percent. The poorest performance at 22.8 percent was on the general floors, and compliance was greatest for staff in the ICU. I found it absolutely disturbing that patients on medical/surgical floors had to endure 30 percent less compliance with a simple safety measure just because they weren't ill enough to be in an intensive care unit.

The April 1999 issue of the *American Journal of Infection Control* published an article titled "Interventions for Improving Hand Washing Compliance." It reported that in September 1997, a hand-washing audit at a Florida hospital revealed only a 27 percent compliance rate. This alarming statistic prompted the institution to assess its guidelines and to increase their surveillance. A second audit conducted a year later showed a little bit of improvement – 39 percent – but not enough to consider its efforts a success. Finally, the results of the audit were made known to the staff, and two subsequent audits showed that people were finally paying attention; cooperation was now between 63 and 74 percent.

These people, especially nurses, are not just being obtuse on this point. There are reasonable explanations for their reluctance to perform this simple task. One, after people have been in this business for a while, their hands tend to be perennially dry and chapped from washing their hands so much, and no lotion in the world really puts the moisture back into their skin. Soap and water simply draw natural oils from the skin when it is used too many times a day. Two, because of the way the system is set up, nurses have to pass from one patient to the next many, many times in a day. They don't have the luxury of staying in one patient's room and attending to every task for that single patient before moving onto another. If they could work this way, they would greatly reduce allow nurses the time to set up a well thought out plan for their patient's care so that they can avoid having to flit from room to room, patient to patient, handing out piecemeal care. Under these conditions, if they were to follow acceptable guidelines, they could be washing their hands every few minutes for hours at a time.

In October 2002, in response to this decades-long dilemma, the CDC issued new guidelines for hand hygiene. Doctors and nurses are now advised to abandon using soap and water unless their hands are actually visibly soiled with blood or other materials, and to start using fast-drying alcohol gels to kill more germs, save time, and simply make it easier for them to keep their hands clean. Staff members can now substitute a half-minute hand washing with soap and water with a 15-second alcohol gel hand rub. A great deal of the time they can now bypass a sink, running water, a bar of soap, paper towels and wet hands. Washing with soap and water is still recommended before and after eating and after using the restroom.

Action Steps

- Don't be afraid to make your expectations on this subject known to your healthcare providers. Many patients are hesitant because they don't want to imply that staff members aren't "clean" or that they aren't conscientious about their duties. You might be intimidated, but there are ways to diffuse the situation. First of all, don't forget that simple courtesy goes a long way. So avoid bringing up the subject in a strident or accusatory voice, and don't insinuate that the staff doesn't already know enough to wash their hands. Instead, make a statement that is non-blaming, while at the same time expresses your concerns. "I can see how busy you all are, and when you feel that you can't do everything, hand washing is probably one of the first things to drop to the bottom of the list. But I know what the statistics are on nosocomial infections (use that word—it will prove that you have done your homework. It is pronounced "know-so-ko-me-ul"), and I want to make sure I don't have to fight the battle of infection as well as the one I'm already in. So I won't feel comfortable unless you wash your hands before you touch my body or anything invasive to it."

- For people who just cannot face a confrontation with a staff member, or those who do not want to keep repeating themselves on this issue, the solution is to tape an eye-catching, easy-to-read sign on the door. We did this in our daughter's room when she was ill. Using colored paper, we wrote "PLEASE WASH YOUR HANDS AND WEAR GLOVES AS APPRO-PRIATE" in large, black letters. You can also post the sign over your bed, but we found that hanging it on the door alerted staff members before they ever reached our daughter. The increase in compliance was so immediate and so dramatic that the infection control specialist made her own signs and placed them on the doors to all the rooms in the pediatric oncology unit. It is much easier to explain to staff members *in advance* that you are aware of the importance of hand washing and that you want them to be extra cautious. You don't have to feel that you are personally pointing the finger at anyone, and the staff knows that you are an informed consumer with high expectations for recovery in a safe environment.

- Know that the CDC recommends a 15-20 second hand washing process when using soap and water. Sing the "Happy Birthday" song to yourself twice as a way to estimate the proper time.

- Be sure that the soap dispensers and paper towel holders in your room are filled because gels are not useful in every situation. Some staff members cannot use them because they are allergic to the alcohol content, and some staff *shouldn't* be using gel because their hands are visibly soiled, and only soap and water will do. Let your nurse know if soap or towels are gone because it's far too easy for staff to skip washing their hands when the materials aren't readily available.

- Observe the location of the paper towel dispenser. The paper towels should not be situated in an area that will potentially expose them to the "splash zone" from the sink. Unfortunately, this is usually exactly where they are located. See if there is a reasonable location that will allow easy access to the towels but prevent them from being splashed by dirty water from the sink. Check to see that towels can be easily removed from the dispenser. Jammed paper towels will cause staff and visitors alike to reach into the dispenser with wet or contaminated hands, thereby contaminating the clean towels.

- Be informed. Staff members need to wash their hands before and after any direct contact with you—including when they start IV lines, before they put gloves on and after they take them off, after they touch contaminated items such as urine-measuring containers, and after they use the restroom. Because hands can be contaminated during glove removal, it is not enough to simply just don a new pair of gloves without washing their hands first.

- Be sure that alcohol gel is available right at your bedside at all times. The hospital should be able to provide it, but to be absolutely certain it's on hand, buy some at the drug store and pack it in your suitcase before you arrive.

- Wash your own hands regularly, and ask all visitors and volunteers to do the same. Disposable towelettes or alcohol gel hand washes are more practical for patients who are not mobile.

- Intact skin provides a significant barrier to infection, so protect yourself by keeping your skin moist and healthy instead of scaly, dry or cracked. Try not to bite your nails or disrupt your cuticles since this may provide a portal for dangerous microbes. Bring hand lotion to the hospital with you, or ask your nurse for some. Hospitals usually have this product available for patients.

- Observe your caregiver's hands to be certain that her skin is intact and has a healthy appearance. Dry, cracked, or flaking skin is more prone to breaking down, and fissures in the skin can harbor bacteria. Of course, if someone's skin gives you doubts, telling him or her about it certainly presents a delicate problem, so it might be easier to have his or her superior discreetly assess the situation.

Nail Polish and Artificial Nails

It was long suspected that nail polish and artificial nails were sources of hospital infections, and recent studies seem to support this hypothesis. In 1997, an Oklahoma City hospital had an outbreak of the bacteria *Pseudomonas*. It affected 46 infants, with 16 of them dying from their infections. Two strains of pseudomonas were isolated from the babies and were found to be present in the hand cultures of three of the nurses. One nurse had long natural fingernails, another had artificial nails, and the third had short natural nails. Information obtained from DNA testing suggested a causal link between the long or artificial nails and the deadly pseudomonas infections, but did not provide a categorical conclusion. So unfortunately, the testing did not offer definitive ammunition for outlawing the use of artificial nails and polish. The authors of the study would only state that requiring short, natural nails was a "reasonable policy that might reduce the incidence of hospital-acquired infections."

Some hospitals are aware of this problem and have rules already in place. But rules that merely stay on the books and aren't put into practice have no teeth. In December 1999, our daughter was hospitalized in a pediatric intensive care unit with a severe case of pneumonia. I noticed that her respiratory therapist had long, red acrylic nails, and she often wore flashy decals on her nails. She was performing duties such as suctioning Kate's ventilator tube and dispensing medication into the ventilator lines. On several occasions, her nails were so long that she actually perforated her gloves with the tips and had to re-glove. When we asked her about them, she simply told us that she was unaware of any hospital policy regarding fingernails. This means that even if the hospital did have a policy against using artificial nails, the therapist didn't know about it, so we were essentially in the same boat we would have been in if there had been no rules at all.

Action Steps

- Educate yourself about the generally accepted recommendations on cleanliness and be specific when speaking to staff. This lets people know that you've done your research, and they're dealing with someone who is more savvy than most about how infections spread.

- Some studies suggest that freshly applied nail polish does not increase the amount of bacteria, but that polish that is chipped or has been worn for longer than four days may contain greater numbers of bacteria. So when you look at someone's painted nails, don't panic. Just check to see that they are pristine and clean. But be particularly vigilant about artificial nails because they appear more likely to harbor organisms, and their very length can make them a hindrance to effective hand washing.

In studies, higher numbers of bacteria have been cultured from artificial nails (both before and after hand washing) than from natural nails because moisture is trapped at the interface between the natural nail and the artificial nail. This could be the cause of the growth of bacteria and fungus.

- The operating room is one place where staff members should avoid the use of nail polish and artificial nails while they're on duty. If you see OR staff members with artificial nails, let them know about the Association of Perioperative Registered Nurses recommendation that "artificial or acrylic nails should not be worn" in the OR setting. You can also tell them about the 1999 *Journal of the American Dental Association* article that urged *all* healthcare workers to refrain from the use of artificial nails.

- Your hospital should have a clear written policy regarding the use of polish and artificial nails in all units, and the information should be disseminated. There ought to be an easy place to reference information when questions or concerns arise. If a policy is in place but staff members are unaware of its existence, it is virtually useless. The National Patient Safety Foundation explains it succinctly when they state that "No policy means that everything is allowed."

- If you are taking care of a loved one at home who uses intravenous devices, a ventilator, or who requires dressing changes for a catheter site or for a wound, adhere to the same standards as the staff in a hospital.

Gloves

In the past two decades, the use of gloves has steadily increased because it's been proven that they provide a barrier to the transmission of HIV and other blood-borne pathogens. In 1987, The CDC began to recommend that healthcare workers wear gloves routinely because of the potential for HIV transmission between patients and their providers. As of April 2002, the CDC has advised workers to wear gloves whenever there is the potential for contact with blood or other bodily fluids, mucous membranes, non-intact skin, items soiled with blood or other bodily fluids, as well as for venipuncture and other vascular access procedures. But patients need to remember that these are *recommendations*, not hard and fast rules, so don't expect religious adherence, and be prepared to quote the CDC when you ask staff members to observe your simple request.

The FDA (Food and Drug Administration – the agency responsible for issuing standards to regulate the quality of latex gloves) relies on standards issued by the American Society for Testing and Materials (ASTM). Defects, such as pinholes, tears, or rips, compromise a glove's ability to act as a barrier, and they present a health risk to both patients and healthcare workers. The current requirements state that gloves cannot be sold for medical uses if leaks are found at rates that exceed 15 defects per 1,000 for surgeon's gloves and 25 defects per 1,000 for patient examination gloves. Surgeon's gloves have more stringent parameters because they contact internal areas of the body and have longer exposure times to blood and bodily fluids. Studies conducted to evaluate the saturation levels of surgical latex gloves suggest that some viruses may penetrate the seemingly intact barrier of a surgical glove. Consequently, surgeons will often "double glove" or, during long procedures, rely on scheduled glove changes to try to ensure that their gloves don't wear out and become prone to tears and leaks. Gloves that are compromised in any way, or ones that become saturated with bodily fluids for long periods of time, may allow for the transmission of pathogens.

The numbers in the above paragraph represent the Acceptable Quality Levels (AQL) for defects in medical gloves. These standards have improved quality, but the numbers themselves imply that a certain amount of flaws are built into the glove supply and we should expect not only holes, but possibly endotoxin contamination and the presence of residual chemicals from the manufacturing process. The reality of acceptable flaws should alert patients to the fact that gloves alone are not going to prevent all cross-contamination.

Action Steps

- Expect perfect adherence to the CDC guidelines for hand hygiene listed above.

- Hospital personnel should wear gloves when there is any risk to a patient, but determining which situations warrant glove use can be a gray area. Hospital policy should stipulate the circumstances under which staff must absolutely wear gloves; however, the staff also has leeway to make their own judgments in other situations. It is your prerogative to request that they wear gloves when you feel it is necessary.

- Gloves are not an alternative to proper hand hygiene, and you must understand that even when double gloving is used, it is not a substitute for hand washing. Since it is virtually impossible to ensure that every glove that contacts a patient is free of defects, it makes hand washing even more critical. Well before they touch you, ask your healthcare workers to wash their hands both before and after wearing gloves.

- Ask your nurse to be sure that a glove size that actually fits his or her hand is readily available in your room. In fact, your room should always be stocked with several sizes since any number of staff members may need to wear gloves around you. This is vitally important since healthcare workers will go to great lengths to avoid putting on a pair of gloves that form an uncomfortable fit. A glove that is too tight is simply annoying, it may restrict blood flow to the fingers, and it is probably more prone to tearing because the latex is exceeding its expansion limits. Gloves that are too small are an accident waiting to happen if someone comes along with long fingernails. And gloves that are too large create significant impairment when a person is trying to perform fine motor tasks such as IV therapy.

- You need to be aware that the Infusion Nurse's Society in Massachusetts is in the forefront of setting strong recommendations for all practices related to intravenous lines, including glove use. The society recommends the use of gloves for *all* infusion procedures—including inserting an IV line, injecting medications into an existing IV line, and removing IV lines. If you are asking personnel to wear gloves and are meeting resistance, tell them about the Infusion Nurse's Society which can be contacted at (781) 440-9408, or have them check the website www.insl.org for current standards. It is also worth mentioning that it sends the message that, when it comes to your healthcare, you think of the ball as being equally in your court.

One last point I want to make on this subject: As a dentist, I know that dentists are at a high risk of cross contamination; in other words, we can give and take germs freely from and to our patients. Since we spend most of the day with our hands in people's mouths, clean, gloved hands are absolutely critical. Dental training involves extensive training in infection control, and one professor made a lasting impression when he showed our class a slide of a used glove that had been scanned by an electron microscope. The surface of the glove looked like a sieve. "Is this what you are going to rely on to protect you and your patients?" he asked. "If you think you don't have to wash your hands *before* and *after* wearing gloves, remember this picture." Granted, this was 1984, before the CDC recommendations and prior to the FDA standards, so glove quality was not as good as it is today. Still, this was an amazingly effective teaching tool since I still remember, to this day, the image he presented us, and I rely on it to reinforce my own dedication to avoid making my hands the source of someone else's infection.

Antibiotics

The discovery of antibiotics—that "magic bullet" for the prevention and treatment of microbial infections—was the genesis of a new age in medicine. Physicians now had simple, effective therapies for serious, even life-threatening, infections. Patients looked at the new wonder drugs as nothing short of miraculous. The term *magic bullet* did indeed seem to fit, for all one had to do was take a pill or get a shot, and the medicine seemed to "understand" exactly what it was supposed to search out and destroy. (However, it must be noted that while antibiotics are "antimicrobial agents," they do not attack *all* microbes, a term that covers a vast territory of bacteria, fungi, and parasites or viruses. Antibiotics kill bacteria *but not viruses*.) In the early days, side effects from antibiotics were usually minimal, and patients became accustomed to their almost instant results.

The efficacy of antibiotic therapy has led to its widespread use and, unfortunately, its misuse. For too long, physicians have prescribed antibiotics "just to be on the safe side," meaning, "I'm not really sure if you need these or not, but I'll give them to you anyway." In addition, patients often insist on having antibiotics at the first sign of illness. A recent study conducted at the Medical College of Georgia suggests that "90 to 95 percent of all infections are viral or low-acuity bacterial infections" which do not need antibiotic therapy. Dr. Jim Wilde of the Medical College of Georgia estimates that less than 10 percent of bronchitis cases may need to be treated with antibiotics and only 10 to 15 percent of sore throats may require drug therapy. Little thought has been given to the long-term consequences of such injudicious use. After all, what harm could it do? "If the infection is caused by bacteria, the patient will improve after a program of antibiotics, and if it's from a virus, it will run its course anyway. It's not as if the antibiotics will do any harm." Or so we thought.

In the United States alone, the CDC estimates that 100 million courses of antibiotics are prescribed each year. Approximately half of these are considered unnecessary because they are prescribed for viral infections, and, as we said, viruses are not affected in the least by antibiotics. The current CDC estimate is that 70 % of the bacteria that routinely cause hospital infections have acquired some resistance to our most commonly used antibiotics. And the big question is: Is this just the tip of the iceberg? Pathogens live by the motto "survival of the fittest" just as much as any other living thing. For pathogens, survival these days means learning to alter their genetic blueprint to resist destruction by antibiotics. Because bacteria are so adept at changing and mutating in response to drug therapy, antibiotic resistance now poses a serious and ongoing threat to our success in treating infectious diseases.

Patients often ask me to prescribe antibiotics for a variety of reasons. When I try to educate them about the dangers of using them when they are not needed, people will invariably say, "That doesn't apply to me because I've only used antibiotics twice in the past five years." What patients fail to realize is that *the bacteria become resistant, not the person.* And when resistant bacteria are surfacing in the population, they will not selectively infect only those individuals who have misused antibiotics. In other words, your neighbor's repeated misuse of antibiotics might be the source of the resistant bacteria that find their way into *your* body. People who use antibiotics at the drop of a hat are actually letting their bodies be used as a training ground for a whole army of bacteria trying to learn how to fight antibiotics more efficiently.

Often, antibiotics are prescribed without any laboratory tests to identify which bacteria is actually the infective organism, so if it doesn't work, it might be because the prescription is treating the wrong bacteria. But that won't be detected until the patient has finished her course of treatment and she reports that she still has not gotten any better. Then again, the patient's condition may not have improved because the microbes are resistant and will not respond to the standard course of treatment. One never knows. This results in a period of prolonged illness and the opportunity to spread the infection to others. When organisms are resistant to our "first-line" (standard) antimicrobial agents, physicians switch to "second-line" drugs. These drugs are often more costly and have to be administered by injection or intravenously instead of orally, thereby increasing the odds of complications and using up even more rapidly diminishing healthcare resources.

The public continues to experience errors on both ends of the antibiotic spectrum. The information given above includes facts about the overuse of antibiotics, but the fact is that under-utilization can be just as dangerous. Certain conditions warrant pre-medication with antibiotics, so ask your doctor about your need for antibiotic coverage (prophylaxis). In April, 2007 The American Heart Association updated the requirements for antibiotic coverage in patients undergoing dental procedures. Antibiotics are recommended for patients with artificial heart valves, those with a history of endocarditis, unrepaired or incompletely repaired cyanotic congenital heart disease, a defect repaired with a prosthetic material or device (within the first six months after placement), a repaired defect with a residual defect near a prosthetic patch or device, and cardiac transplants that develop a problem in a heart valve. The major change is that individuals with conditions including heart murmurs, mitral valve prolapse, rheumatic heart disease, aortic stenosis, ventricular and atrial septal defects, pacemakers, defibrillators, stents, and bypass patients are *no longer advised* to have routine coverage with antibiotics before dental visits. And it is important to know that maintaining excellent oral hygiene is thought to offer protection from infection by reducing the numbers of bacteria that can be introduced into the bloodstream via the oral cavity. Speak to your physician and to your dentist about your specific situation.

Action Steps

- You need to change your mindset about antibiotics immediately. Don't think of them as a harmless addition to any course of treatment; think of them as serious medications to be used only when medically necessary.

- Never pressure your physician to prescribe antibiotics unless there is a clear indication that they are needed. If you insist on antibiotics you don't need, you will naturally attribute your improvement over the next few days to their effectiveness when, in reality, you would have improved anyway. This reinforces the erroneous idea that antibiotics are appropriate for every cough, fever, or sore throat, which are usually the manifestations of viral illness. Remember, *antibiotics have no effect on viral infections, only bacterial infections.* We have become a nation of people who expect instant results. We are inundated with advertising that encourages us to utilize medication for every malady. Many illnesses, especially viral infections, simply need to run their course, and time and treatment of symptoms are the best medicine.

- Do not self-medicate with antibiotics that you didn't finish off from a previous illness or that belong to someone else. Do not purchase antibiotics without a prescription at a foreign pharmacy or off the Internet because "they're always good to have around." I see many patients who report that their tooth hurts and then choose to treat the problem with antibiotics left over at home or borrowed some from someone else. Often, the patient does not have an infection at all or the antibiotic he is using is not particularly successful for dental infections.

- If you are prescribed antibiotics, be sure to finish the entire amount, even if the symptoms decrease. Discontinuing the antibiotics when you "start to feel better" only increases the odds that your infection won't be completely eradicated, and you will have to start treatment all over again from the beginning. Partial treatment wounds the microbes, but it doesn't kill them, and it only encourages them to mutate and be more resistant. Remember, if friends and relatives offer to share their leftover antibiotics with you, it only means that they did not complete their entire dose!

- Check with your physician before and after any surgical procedures to see if you truly need antibiotic "prophylaxis." Questions to ask include: "Do I have any risk factors that may increase my odds of developing an infection?" "Do I need to be pre-medicated with antibiotics?" "Why or why not?" "Are you following the American Heart Associations established recommendations for pre-medicating patients with my condition?" If you find out that you are at risk, check with your doctor before you have any procedures that could introduce bacteria into your bloodstream, even something as seemingly harmless as a dental cleaning or ear piercing.

- Conditions that may place you in a high-risk category during dental procedures and warrant a discussion with your physician include prosthetic heart valves, previous endocarditis, shunts, serious congenital heart conditions, and prosthetic joints within two years of placement.

- You may not have a medical condition that predisposes you to infection, but your surgical procedure could be one that potentially carries a greater risk. Be aware of the surgeries with the potential to pose a higher risk of infection: organ transplants, coronary artery grafts, tonsillectomy, colon, gastric or bowel surgery, gallbladder surgery and some cesarean sections. Ask your doctor if your surgery carries any additional risk for infection and ask if you should have antibiotic prophylaxis.

- The American Heart Association is the recognized authority on pre-medication standards, so call them at 1-800-242-8721 or check their website www.americanheart.org for information on guidelines.

As is often the case in healthcare, we are now in the position of being reactive rather than proactive. Instead of dealing with a problem in its infancy, we wait until it reaches a crisis level before we alert the public and begin searching for solutions. This is the situation we are now facing with antibiotic resistance. We hear about the new "super-bugs," and everyone looks to the development of newer, stronger antibiotics, to fight them. Most of us just assume that there are new miracle drugs on the horizon and we expect drug companies to concoct some before the next epidemic hits. But even if a new antibiotic does hit the market in the nick of time, we will eventually succumb to the same fate with new antibiotics that we have with the old if we do not change our usage patterns.

Surveillance

In 1988, the CDC defined surveillance as, "the ongoing, systematic collection, analysis, and interpretation of health data essential to the planning, implementation, and evaluation of public health practice, closely integrated with the timely dissemination of these data to those who need to know." In a hospital, surveillance includes observing staff to see that they are in compliance with the rules about infection control, safety, and overall patient care. This is important because strict adherence to certain infection control actions have been directly tied to a better optimum survival rate for patients. It takes highly trained personnel to monitor the staff and keep an eye on patient outcomes on a consistent basis. Just spot-checking isn't good enough because for every problem identified, a hundred will be missed. Overall, surveillance is important in a hospital because it helps spot those small, subtle sources of infection before they blow up into a huge outbreak. In fact, more than 90 percent of hospital infections do not occur in recognized outbreaks or epidemics.

Without a commitment to regular surveillance, we lose the opportunity to recognize the true extent of hospital infections, to search for innovative ways to prevent them, and to identify new trends in disease patterns. With nosocomial infections claiming 90,000 lives per year, and 25 percent of all doctor visits now involving possible infectious disorders like influenza, sinus infections, pneumonia or strep throat, the threat to public health from dangerous pathogens shows no signs of abating. Given that the risks are increasing, it is disappointing that 30 years of hospital surveillance activities in the United States have yet to produce a systematic, universally accepted methodology for evaluating hospital acquired infections, virtually guaranteeing that significant numbers of infections will be overlooked. Studies conducted *over 20 years ago* by the CDC proved that surveillance by qualified infection control personnel reduces the occurrence of nosocomial infections. The CDC recommends that all healthcare organizations have a system in place for the surveillance, prevention and control of hospital infections.

The CDC says that data should be disseminated to those who "need to know." Informed patients have a distinct advantage over any member of the staff in a certain sense: they are a captive audience, and as such, can serve as the eyes and ears of the Infection Control Professionals (ICP). ICP's establish baseline infection rates, identify outbreaks of infection, evaluate infection control measures, educate staff members about ways to identify and prevent infection, and reinforce staff members' compliance with infection control guidelines. They determine when and where infective organisms are surfacing in the institution and look for trends in antibiotic resistance. They obtain information about possible infections and resistant organisms from staff members, from reviewing lab results, from medical records, and from monitoring physician orders for antibiotics—but rarely from patients themselves. Obviously, these are extraordinarily important tasks, but ICPs cannot be everywhere. Patients can be adjuncts to their hospital's built-in surveillance program.

Action Steps

- Do you know if your institution has a full-time Infection Control Practitioner on staff? Smaller hospitals may not have a full-time staff member, but all should at least have part-time staff available for surveillance. If you have any questions about infection control or suspect that you have an infection, ask for a consultation with the individual responsible for monitoring infection rates.

- Be aware of the need for constant diligence regarding infection control practices. No one can afford to be complacent since a single overlooked step can be the action that results in a life-threatening infection.

- You don't have to be an expert, but you need to be somewhat informed on this subject so you can intelligently evaluate the quality of the infection control practices utilized in your hospital. After reading this chapter, you will know the infection control measures to look for and possess the ability to form a valid assessment of the staff's competence in these matters.

- Reinforce patient care practices by tactfully reminding staff members about safety measures that appear to be lacking, and practice your own infection control methods, such as good hand washing.

- As an adjunct to the professionals, your job is to provide feedback, both positive and negative, to the hospital staff and to the administration about the infection control efforts you observe. Speaking to them directly at the time of your hospitalization is preferred, but don't discount the value of writing a letter after you return home or making a phone call. You may have noticed a flaw in the system that is endangering other patients and your comments could save someone's life. "A nurse with a cold was leaning directly over a patient and not wearing a mask." "The bathroom and surfaces of my room were visibly dirty." "All the soap dispensers I saw were empty."

- ICPs are always asking: "What organisms are causing infection? Is there a cluster or a pattern? In what units are the problems occurring? Do we have any infections in which first-line antibiotics are not proving effective? This means there is a resistant organism in the hospital." You may actually be of service in helping ICPs discover the answers to these questions. If you are told that you have an infection, insist that you become part of the statistics. The ICP should be notified so that any pertinent information about your case can be included in their report.

- You and your family will be valuable additions to a hospital's surveillance program if you know what to look for and where to report your observations. Is your room clean? Is the house-keeping staff keeping your floor and bathroom clean? Does your room have soap and paper towels at all times? Are staff members washing their hands and wearing gloves as appropriate? If you are told that you have an infection, does it meet the criteria to be classified as a nosocomial infection? Why or why not? Is your infection part of an outbreak or cluster of infections? Will your infection be counted as part of the hospital's nosocomial infection rate? Why or why not? The staff members who can provide these answers and who are interested in your observations include your nurse, the charge nurse, infection control personnel, and the hospital administrator. No one is more interested in keeping you safe in the hospital than YOU are—so be sure to ask every question and don't be satisfied until you have every answer and explanation you need.

- Realize that with the almost immediate release of medical patients after invasive surgeries, your hospital-acquired infection may not be diagnosed until after you have been released from the hospital. Infections that may have originated in the hospital are being diagnosed by home health nurses or by physicians in their offices, and patients who are treated on an outpatient basis without readmission to the hospital will not have their infections counted in the hospital's nosocomial infection rate. If you suspect that your infection originated in the hospital, phone the hospital's infection control specialists to alert them to the facts. Ask the infection control staff person to phone your doctor for more information, to investigate thoroughly the potential sources of the infection, to add an entry to your medical record documenting your infection, and to let you know of their findings.

Surface Disinfection

The *Chicago Tribune* series "Unhealthy Hospitals" reported that since 1995, a significant number of U.S. hospitals have been cited for violations involving cleanliness and sanitation. Surface disinfection is an important step in the infection control process, but one that is often overlooked. Over the years, I have been alarmed by the almost non-existent disinfection practices in hospitals and other healthcare settings. Surface disinfection has a dual benefit: it helps protect patients from hospital-acquired infections, and it maintains a safe work environment for employees.

Cleaning and disinfecting are not interchangeable terms. "Cleaning" refers to the physical removal of organic materials from surfaces. "Disinfection" refers to the use of a product to kill or inactivate disease-causing pathogens on inanimate objects *after* the surface has been cleaned. Basic cleaning followed by disinfection of even potentially contaminated surfaces should be done on a daily basis or more often if needed.

Disinfectants are classified as low, intermediate, or high-level solutions and must be used with strict adherence to the manufacturer's recommendations, which usually require the liquid to remain in contact with a surface for a number of minutes. Many people don't know this, but when they spray the disinfectant on, and then immediately wipe it off with a paper towel, it may not have worked at all. Even if it is left on the appropriate amount of time for the disinfectant to be effective, organic materials, which block its contact with the surface, must be removed ahead of time. Consequently, surface cleaning is always a vital precursor to the disinfection process.

Areas should be disinfected whenever there is a potential for high concentrations of bacteria on a surface or the possibility they can be spread to others. We know that some strains of bacteria can live on environmental surfaces for hours and even days at a time, so cleaning and disinfecting must be an ongoing process if the public is to be afforded the greatest protection. The *Chicago Tribune* reported that since 1995, federal inspectors have cited 31 Chicago hospitals for failure to sanitize rooms properly in between patients. The reality is that your supposedly "clean" room could be functioning as a large petri dish.

It has been estimated that 20 to 40 percent of all nosocomial infections caused by contact transmission come directly from the hands of healthcare workers. The hands of hospital personnel, through direct patient contact or contact with contaminated surfaces, pick up potentially dangerous organisms, which are then transmitted to medical devices or directly to wounds. A three-year outbreak of fungal infections in a newborn ICU in New Hampshire was attributed to healthcare workers who were transmitting a fungus from their pet dogs to the infants via their contaminated hands. A 1999 article by Pittet, et al. in *The Archives of Internal Medicine* confirmed that the type of service being provided the patient (whether it was invasive or superficial) and the duration of patient contact both influenced hand contamination. Each minute of patient contact added more colony forming units (CFU) of bacteria to the hands of healthcare workers. Not all contact causes the same danger however. Respiratory care results in a greater degree of hand contamination than contact with body fluid secretions, and contact with body secretions causes more contamination than contact with a patient's intact skin. Healthcare personnel should not be nonchalant about touching their patients without hand washing or wearing gloves, because we know that significant hand contamination is occurring at the microscopic level.

Which surfaces have the potential for transmitting pathogens? Surfaces that sustain the most traffic. Consider the number of hands that contact door handles, telephones, bathroom surfaces, bed controls, toys in waiting rooms and playrooms and intravenous pumps. Items such as blood pressure cuffs, thermometers and pulse oximeters (devices to measure the oxygen saturation in the bloodstream) often travel from room to room. Even stethoscopes have been cultured and found to be a possible vector for pathogens. A 1997 article in *Infection Control and Hospital Epidemiology* reported that the contaminated handle of a shared ear thermometer was the probable cause of hospital-acquired infections involving seven patients. A recent article in the *American Journal of Infection Control* stated that the potentially deadly bacteria *Pseudomonas aeruginosa*, a common culprit in nosocomial infections, may survive in water for more than 300 days and on dry hospital floors for as long as 35 days. A 2001 article in *Reuters Medical News* stated that even the materials used in hospital privacy curtains "can serve as reservoirs for fungi that cause nosocomial infections." Most of these surfaces are easy to clean – cheap and simple – so why aren't we doing it?

Action Steps

- Be prepared to clean and disinfect your own room. This may sound like something only a "neat freak" would do, but under these circumstances, it's not an extraordinary measure. During our daughter's many hospitalizations, I observed surfaces being touched by a number of staff members for days on end. Nobody ever disinfected anything. Out of pure concern, I began bringing my own disinfectants to the hospital to wipe down the many contaminated surfaces. As a dentist, I had greater access to hospital-level disinfectants than the general public, but anyone can bring in products such as Lysol, alcohol, or peroxide. Or better yet, visit your local home healthcare supply store or shop online for solutions that provide hospital-level surface disinfection. Many reasonably priced disinfection products are packaged as disposable cloths in plastic containers that can be easily transported to the hospital.

- If you have questions about any germicidal product, contact the EPA (Environmental Protection Agency) for guidance. Their website is www.epa.gov.

- Ask your nurse or infection control specialist to provide you with a disinfection product and instruct you how to use it. For example, you might need to wear gloves because it could be irritating to your skin, or the substance might need to sit on the surface, wet, for a few minutes in order to work. You are not helpless; you can play an important role in keeping yourself or loved ones safe.

- Identify the surfaces that should be disinfected:

  1. Door handles
  2. Sink and toilet handles
  3. IV pumps
  4. Stethoscopes
  5. Phones
  6. Bed controls and TV remote
  7. Blood pressure cuffs
  8. Portable thermometers
  9. Curtains (Ask that visibly stained or soiled curtains be replaced with a freshly laundered pair.)

- If blood, urine, feces, vomitus or any bodily fluid contaminates the floor of your room, have the nurse call housekeeping immediately to clean *and* disinfect the area.

- Encourage your hospital to use disposable cloths for cleaning the floors and plastic mops that can be wiped down with a disinfectant before each use. If traditional mops are still being used, ask if the mop is clean, if the water is fresh, and if an appropriate germicide has been added to it. I can't tell you the number of times janitorial staff entered my daughter's room with a bucket of brown, filthy-looking water and a dirty mop to "clean" the floors. I would take one look at the water and ask them to refrain from mopping. A nurse once insisted that the floors had to be cleaned, and to placate me, she told the housekeeping staff member to dispose of the dirty water and use clean water. Unfortunately, as I reminded her, the bucket and the mop were already contaminated with potentially lethal pathogens, and clean water was not going to improve the situation. Don't let anyone with a bucket of filthy water used in 20 other rooms mop your floor!

- Ask if your hospital trains the housekeeping staff about the importance of infection control measures. The hospital housekeeping staff is not cleaning a hotel room, which just needs to *look* clean and tidy. Actions by the housekeeping staff can cause or prevent life-threatening infections—and time must be allotted for thorough training.

- Make sure your nurses and doctors wipe the round end of the stethoscope that will be touching your skin with an alcohol wipe. The stethoscope touches dozens of bodies a day and has been shown to be a potential source of shared germs.

- Ask that a plastic blood pressure cuff be used and be sure that it is wiped down with disinfectant before and after use. If you at an increased risk for infection, ask for a plastic cuff to be left at your bedside, to be used exclusively for you.

- Steer your children away from the toys in waiting rooms and play areas. It is only common sense that these items are teeming with bacteria from being touched by dozens of kids and even placed into children's mouths. Often these items are not cleaned at all or only sporadically. Get in the routine of bringing a book from home and reading to your child while waiting to be seen by the doctor.

Communicable Diseases from Roommates, Staff, or Anyone Else Who Enters the Room

Hospital-acquired illnesses run the gamut from simple cold viruses passed from one patient to another, to devastating bloodstream infections from a surgeon who is unaware that he is a chronic carrier of staph bacteria. Communicable diseases can be spread throughout a hospital by staff members who are ill, by people who are "carriers" of bacteria but asymptomatic themselves, and by those individuals just coming down with an illness and aren't aware that they are contagious. Incredibly, the spouses, children, and even the pets of healthcare workers have been identified as sources for the pathogens that prey on hospitalized patients.

No matter how nice your roommate might be, he or she is another source of pathogens that can make you sick. Most people prefer a single hospital room for privacy considerations, but it also offers protection against hospital-acquired infections. A roommate who is hacking away with a cough should obviously be avoided, but other signs of a problem may not be so easy to identify. You will also be exposed to your roommate's visitors and their germs, so good hand washing is a necessity for everyone entering your room, and proper surface disinfection is especially vital. Again, a brightly colored sign is a way to let everyone know, without confrontation, how important this measure is.

A 1998 study published in the medical journal *Infection Control and Hospital Epidemiology* showed that the bacteria *Bordetella pertussis* and Respiratory Syncytial Virus (RSV) were present in the air of the rooms of over 50 percent of pediatric patients with RSV and Pertussis (whooping cough). The RSV was detected as far as seven meters away from the patient's bedside and for as long as seven days. All of the children above were in private rooms, but nevertheless, they were potentially contagious to everyone on the floor. And let's not forget the risk to the subsequent occupants if these rooms are not meticulously cleaned and disinfected between patients. It is easy to see how the nature of pathogens and the diagnosis of the patients around you can be the source of your nosocomial infection.

Patients are generally aware that their caregivers can be a source of germs, but they may never have considered the risk of communicable diseases from roommates, visitors, and volunteers or thought about the actions they can take to minimize their chances of experiencing a debilitating setback.

Action Steps

- Any patient, and especially those at an increased risk of infection, can request a private room.

- Patients who must share a room need to ask discreetly if their roommate's condition poses any additional risk of infection.

- All visitors and volunteers need to wash their hands and postpone visits if they are ill.

- Know that recent studies have suggested that visitors should refrain from touching or sitting on the patient's bed. Visitors can bring germs from outside the hospital and deposit them on the patient's bedding, thereby potentially exposing the patient to additional pathogens. Be sure your visitors have a chair to sit on.

- Hospitals should have established policies in place to protect patients from communicable diseases, and policies should exist for situations that pose risks to patients. Examples include employee illness, the use of fingernail polish and artificial nails, glove usage, and a protocol for surfaces that need to be disinfected daily (sinks, floors, IV pumps, door handles, bed rails, etc.)

Intravenous Lines

It is estimated that between 33 and 48 percent of hospital acquired infections are related to intravenous devices. Intravenous lines (also called IVs or catheters) function as direct pipelines into your bloodstream, which is of great benefit when delivering medications, but potentially lethal when delivering unwelcome pathogens. Lack of hand washing, a staff member who is rushed, and improper technique are just a few of the errors that can transform the plastic tubing we rely on to deliver life-saving medications into a source of life-threatening infections. The CDC reports that approximately 400,000 potential catheter-related bloodstream infections occur each year with a mortality rate of 10 to 20 percent. The care and maintenance of your intravenous line is your nurse's responsibility, but you can significantly reduce your chance of being one of the above statistics.

Periodically, nurses have to reprogram an IV pump, but sometimes she or he is scheduled to come in precisely when the patient is being wheeled out of the room for X-rays or other tests. You do not want to find yourself waiting in the hallway for an X-ray with your IV pump alarm going off because the medication dose has been infused and the pump is waiting for the flush to be delivered. We went through many incidents where staff members ferrying our daughter around for a test would have to place her pump on hold every few minutes so the alarm would stop beeping. This would sometimes go on for extended periods of time, and it virtually guaranteed that she did not receive her entire dose of medication on time. I remember thinking that alarms were well designed to be loud and irritating for good reason: to alert someone to a problem and attract immediate attention. One day, as we waited in the hallway, the alarm began to escalate in frequency because it had been placed on hold so many times. It was beginning to upset Kate, so I placed it on hold myself. Then, during the sonogram procedure, the technician placed the pump on hold again, and so did the transport person who took us back to the room. In the course of 30 minutes, five people had touched the keypad of the IV pump with their unwashed hands. As soon as we were inside Kate's room, I wiped down the entire pump with my antiseptic spray. But most patients would never even realize that their pump had just been heavily contaminated with an array of germs, germs that could easily be introduced into an IV line as the nurse touches the keypad and then injects medication into the tubing.

It might be annoying to have one's lunch or nap interrupted so the IV line and pump can be reprogrammed before the patient is removed from a room, but there are worse things than feeling pestered. Many intravenous medications have very specific protocols dictating how many minutes the infusion needs to run, the rate at which the drug is to enter the person's bloodstream, and the need for a flush to ensure that all the fluid has been pushed through the tubing and out the other end. Every attempt should be made to minimize interrupting this protocol when sending a patient off the floor for an indeterminate amount of time.

Action Steps

- Be aware that the first step in proper IV insertion is always for staff members to wash their hands *and* to put on gloves.

- Don't let anyone start an IV in your arm without first prepping the skin with alcohol or betadine or both. Do not let anybody stick your unwashed flesh with a needle.

- Ideally, only gloved fingers should touch your skin to feel for your veins. Many nurses and technicians prepped our daughter's skin and then removed their glove to feel for the vein with their ungloved finger for greater tactile sensation. (Children's veins can be difficult to access.) When we told personnel that we wanted them to prep Kate's skin again before the venipuncture, they often became defensive or flustered, even though they were obviously aware that their bare fingers could potentially contaminate the "clean" area where the IV was to be inserted. It is understandable that technicians need to un-glove for some procedures, but make sure they take the time to prep their hands again before penetration of the needle. Vigilance here is everything.

- Avoid awkward situations by announcing your concerns to the staff well in advance of the start of the procedure. One could offer: "We are very concerned about the possibility of infection, so we routinely ask everyone to wash their hands and wear gloves for all vascular procedures." Stating your goals for venipuncture up front will result in safer catheter usage and less need for an uncomfortable confrontation. Don't wait for staff members to breach protocol and *then* pounce on them. I always found it useful to put the onus on me by saying "I just won't feel comfortable unless everyone wears gloves." No one feels attacked and certainly the staff will not be inclined to deny your request and purposely make you uncomfortable.

- It has been shown that pathogens can adhere to plastic IV tubing, so there are guidelines regarding the number of days that tubing can be used before it must be changed; the standard interval is 72 hours. At the time your IV is started, be sure that a staff member places a sticker on the IV tubing indicating when it is to be replaced. Some institutions write down a "started on" date and others list a "change on" date. Either way, be sure the instructions are obvious. Don't rely on the staff's memory because it can easily be forgotten or on a note in the chart because they don't always look. Be sure that the staff labels the IV tubing with a sticker and that they pay attention to be sure the tubing is changed on the correct day.

- IV pumps are equipped with alarms to beep for a variety of reasons—and every one of them requires prompt attention. Various reasons can be: the machine may not be plugged in and is running on its battery (you want your pump plugged into a wall circuit because it will preserve the battery life for the times when you need to be away from your room); the dose of medication is completely delivered and it's time for a flush (a flush is a small infusion of a saline solution through the IV tubing to ensure that all the medication has been pushed though the tubing and into the patient's bloodstream); the tubing may have an air bubble inside and it has to be purged.

- When the IV pump alarms, be prompt about notifying your nurse with your call button or via a representative. We used to think that we were being "good patients" by not "bothering" the nurse when the IV pump would alarm. If we waited long enough, the nurse would eventually hear the alarm or she might happen to come into the room for another reason. Eventually, though, we learned to speak up. Whenever a pump alarms, it immediately stops the infusion, and you don't want your IV line to remain static (not running or flowing) for any length of time because a static line can result in a clot at the tip of the catheter and cause a patient to need a new line inserted—a procedure that serves no purpose but to provide another opportunity for infection.

- If you will be leaving your room for X-rays or other tests, ask your nurse if your appointment time will conflict with important medication dosing schedules or the flush after an infusion ends. In the morning, inquire about your plan for the day. If you are going to be transported out of your room, ask that it not interfere with the infusion of important medications such as antibiotics, which must be administered at specific intervals and require a flush procedure afterwards.

- When staff continuously place your IV pump alarm on hold, it also means that a greater number of potentially unwashed hands will contaminate your medical equipment. Insist that the problem with your line be addressed as soon as possible.

- Be sure that the IV pump is set at a minimum "keep open" infusion rate. The "keep vein open" rate or KVO is a minimum infusion rate that should guarantee that your IV line will remain open, or patent, and not clot.

- Let the staff know that you are not in favor of placing the pump on hold for any length of time if it is going to prevent you from receiving your entire dose of medication at the proper interval.

Urinary Catheters

Urinary catheters, also referred to as Foley catheters, are devices used to drain the bladder of urine when the patient is not mobile enough to get up and walk to the bathroom. As long as it is still enclosed in the patient's urinary tract, urine is sterile and harmless; however, it can easily be infected when in contact with bacteria from an outside source, including the patient's own skin or genitalia, the hands of a healthcare worker, or tubing that has been contaminated from improper handling.

Too often, inserting a catheter is looked upon as a routine procedure, yet it should be seen as a last resort, especially if the patient is conscious and able to walk to the bathroom unassisted. And urinary catheters are not a solution for routine incontinence, even though they are sometimes treated that way when there isn't enough staff to see patients safely to the bathroom. If the use of a catheter is unavoidable, the duration of use should be as short as possible.

Amazingly, studies have shown that physicians often forget that their patients are catheterized, and they don't write timely orders to discontinue their use. This is not an innocuous mistake, since each additional day of catheterization presents a greater risk of a urinary tract infection. Even one day can make a difference when a catheter is in place, so patients should not sit back and just wait for someone to remove it. In fact, prompt removal is so important that hospitals are trying out automatic reminder systems for physicians. Every two days, the doctor is reminded to check if a urinary catheter is still medically indicated for a patient. In hospitals where no such system is in place, patients and their loved ones have to function as a kind of low-tech, personal reminder system. Patients themselves need to realize that catheters are an invasive medical device with inherent risks.

People who have contracted UTIs (urinary tract infections) are far more likely to incur other complications stemming from the urinary tract, such as kidney or blood stream infections.

Action Steps

- There should be a real decision-making process before catheterization. In other words, it should not just be employed on a routine basis. Unless it is absolutely necessary, avoid it, and if it is necessary, discontinue it as soon as possible. If you have a broken leg, you might find it a little exasperating to haul yourself into the bathroom, but it is well worth the effort if you consider that it might be preventing a blood clot or infection.

- Urinary catheter insertion must be done under sterile conditions. The skin needs to be prepped several times with an antiseptic such as betadine, the staff member needs to wear sterile gloves (they come sealed in their own package), a sterile, single-use package of lubricant is needed, and a sterile paper drape is needed under the catheter insertion site. A commode next to your bed might be a reasonable compromise between being catheterized and walking unassisted to the bathroom.

- The use of condom-like catheters for men may be associated with a lower risk of UTI, so ask your physician if this is an option. They come in several sizes, so be sure that yours fits comfortably.

- For unconscious or sedated female patients, more than one staff member is needed for proper catheter insertion because it is impossible to hold a patient's legs correctly while still maintaining a sterile field.

- Be sure the catheter is securely taped or strapped to your leg so it will not move out of position and need to be reinserted—yet another potential source of infection.

- Urine should flow only one way in the catheter tubing, so the bag needs to be placed lower than the patient's bladder so gravity can help it flow downward. When patients are transported in their beds, the bag is often placed on top of the bed so it will not become tangled in the wheels. Be sure that the bag is moved back to a low position as soon as possible.

- As with IV lines, you don't want a "static" line where urine is not draining, or worse yet, is backing up into the bladder (urine reflux). This can cause a urinary tract infection, so ask your nurse to show you or your advocate how to manipulate the tubing to drain urine into the bag. It is very simple.

- If the bag appears full, notify the nurse so it can be measured (they need to be sure you're not eliminating more fluid than you're taking in) and emptied.

- For patients catheterized from three to 14 days, antibiotic therapy or "prophylaxis" may be beneficial in preventing a UTI. Ask your physician if this is appropriate.

- Communication with the physician about the necessity, the duration, and the type of catheter is also essential. Ask if you need a catheter coated with a type of silver alloy to reduce the risk of UTIs or a urine drainage bag equipped with an anti-reflux device to prevent urine back-flow into the bladder. If you have previously had a UTI or you have a compromised immune system, these features are even more important to consider.

Surgical Site Infections

Each of the 27 million people who have surgery each year in this country is at risk of developing a life-threatening surgical site infection (SSI). The CDC reports that approximately 500,000 of these occur each year, making them the second most frequently reported hospital-acquired infection behind urinary tract infections. Approximately 15 percent of all hospital infections originate in a surgical site. Aside from the obvious burden of additional pain and suffering for the patient, infections arising from invasive surgical procedures add seven to nine days to the average hospital stay and cost thousands, sometimes even hundreds of thousands of dollars, in additional healthcare expenses. In our daughter's case, the 1997 hospital bill for Kate's nosocomial infection that led to toxic shock syndrome totaled $396,000 for a six-week stay! I often wondered why our insurance company was not outraged by this unnecessary expense.

The reality is that some of the strategies used to prevent surgical site infections will always be out of the patient's control. For instance, your surgeon's operating technique, the quality and temperature of air in the operating room, and the duration and quality of the staff's hand scrub are not areas in which you can expect to have much impact beyond inquiring about them. This aside, there are many basic facts about SSIs that patients need to be aware of and simple strategies that can be used to reduce significantly the odds of developing an infection as a result of a surgical procedure.

Action Steps

- Inform yourself about which factors increase the risk of developing a surgical site infection. Examples are diabetes, nicotine use, malnutrition, obesity, chronic steroid use, prolonged preoperative hospitalization, the presence of the bacteria Staphylococcus aureus in your nostrils (approximately 20 to 30 percent of all healthy adults have asymptomatic nasal colonization with staph), a surgery of long duration, and a reduced immune response due to HIV.

- If your surgeon determines that antibiotic prophylaxis is indicated after an operation, there are three crucial factors to consider. One, you must receive the correct antibiotic, which needs to be effective against the pathogens most commonly associated with the wound infection that most often occurs after your particular surgery. Two, the antibiotic should generally be given intravenously at just the right time to ensure that the peak concentration of the drug will be present in your tissues for the entire duration of the procedure. Most recent recommendations are that antibiotics should be given within 60 minutes before the initial incision. Due to the number of surgeries that do not begin on time, doctors often choose to administer antibiotics via a patient's IV line right in the operating room. Three, there is debate about the need to provide antibiotic therapy after surgery, but if prophylactic antibiotics are to be continued after the procedure they should be stopped within 24 hours, because longer courses of therapy do not appear to reduce SSI rates and may even increase the numbers of organisms resistant to antibiotics. Antibiotics given for known infections or as a part of your overall treatment plan will be continued. The recommendation to stop antibiotics within 24 hours only applies to those antibiotics given as a precaution against infection from the surgery itself.

- Inquire about using a pre-surgical body wash containing chlorhexidine gluconate. Many surgeons are now having their patients bathe the night before their surgery with an anti-microbial body wash to lower the bacterial count on their skin.

- If you are a diabetic, realize that there is a causal relationship between hyperglycemia (high glucose levels) and increased SSIs, especially during the first 48 hours after surgery. Careful control of blood glucose levels before and after surgical procedures is a necessity.

- If the area to be operated on requires hair removal, you need to know that shaving the operative site within 24 hours of the surgery with a razor is associated with significantly higher infection rates than the use of a cream hair remover, or no hair removal at all. One study reported infection rates of 5.6 percent for patients undergoing shaving versus 0.6 percent for patients who had hair removed with a depilatory. The reason is that shaving the skin with a razor can cause small cuts in the skin that provide bacteria a perfect environment to multiply, so clipping the hair is a safer alternative to shaving. If hair removal is unavoidable, your safest bet is for the staff to use clippers immediately before the start of your procedure.

- Be aware that the CDC recommends that sterile gloves and sterile technique be used when changing the dressings on *all* surgical incisions.

- Make a valid attempt to stop using tobacco products before any scheduled surgeries since the use of tobacco causes arterial vasoconstriction, which reduces blood flow to the areas trying to heal and is associated with prolonged healing times.

- Do not leave the hospital without clear instructions regarding the care of your incision and a list of the symptoms to watch for that may indicate that a post-operative infection is present. Remember that it is vital to report these infections so that the right people will be informed of the true scope of the problem of infections in their hospital. If you develop an infection in or around your incision, be sure it gets reported to the hospital staff member who collects data on infections.

- Recent studies have shown a possible correlation between the use of oxygen after surgery and a reduced rate of SSIs. In a study of 500 patients who had colorectal surgery, those who received oxygen during their surgery, and for up to two hours after surgery, had fewer infections. Ask your surgeon if this could helpful to you; it is unlikely that it would be harmful.

- Inquire about the newly FDA-approved antibacterial sutures. These vicryl (dissolving) sutures are coated with Triclosan, an antibacterial agent useful in fighting staphylococcus, the leading cause of surgical site infections. They can be used in areas of soft tissue, but not in cardiac, neurological or ophthalmic procedures.

- Know that keeping warm is now considered an important method to reduce post-operative infection. The patient's temperature should be kept above 36 degrees Celsius as this increases circulation and brings more white blood cells to the area. Ask for a warming blanket if you feel cold or are shivering after surgery.

Ventilator-Associated Pneumonia

Pneumonias that develop as a result of the use of a ventilator brought in to assist breathing are a leading cause of death among patients in intensive care units. The Institute for Healthcare Improvement states that 15 percent of all patients on ventilators will develop pneumonia (called VAP or Ventilator-Associated Pneumonia). It is, in fact, among the most lethal of hospital-acquired infections, with approximately 50 percent of all cases resulting in the patient's death. A majority of nosocomial bacterial pneumonias are attributed to the aspiration of oropharyngeal (mouth and throat) and gastric (stomach) secretions that have been contaminated with harmful bacteria. The actual physical presence of the breathing tube reduces the body's natural defenses against aspiration, along with the fact that the patient is already immobile and heavily sedated. While ventilator-related pneumonia will always present a serious risk for patients, providing the public with basic knowledge about the current recommendations for preventing these infections is an essential component of any comprehensive plan for reducing the high mortality rate associated with this complication.

Action Steps

- Know your susceptibility. Patients who may be at increased risk for ventilator-associated pneumonia are patients who have experienced head or neck trauma, emergency intubations, severe underlying heart, lung, kidney or neurological disease and those having a suppressed immune system.

- Know the risk factors for pneumonia that occur during ventilator use, including being in a continuous supine position (lying flat), having breathing tubes in the nasal cavity instead of the throat, being re-intubated, undergoing frequent ventilator tubing changes, going through a long duration of ventilation, the development of gastrointestinal bleeding from stress ulcers, the use of paralyzing medications, the development of blood clots and the lack of routine cleaning of the oral cavity.

- Realize that preventive antibiotic prophylaxis is often not indicated for routine use in ventilated patients, although there is some disagreement in the literature about its effectiveness in preventing VAP. The use of antibiotics can reduce the number of dangerous bacteria in the patient's body, but using antibiotics as a matter of course may lead to resistant organisms that are even more dangerous. Ask your doctor about your loved one's need for antibiotic therapy.

- If a patient is on a ventilator, elevating the bed to 30 to 45 degrees (as opposed to lying flat or supine position) is thought to decrease the chance of aspiration, a risk factor for pneumonia. This may not be appropriate for patients with Acute Respiratory Distress Syndrome (ARDS) who may need to lay flat to increase their oxygenation.

- Preventing blood clots will lessen a patient's chances of developing VAP, so ask what actions and/or medications will be used to stop clots.

- "Sedation Breaks" in which the patient is brought to a higher level of consciousness to see if they can breath on their own are important, so bring it up to the staff. Some studies recommend a "daily trial of weaning" to identify the earliest opportunity to remove the patient from the ventilator.

- Care of the oral cavity, nasal passages and lips are now considered part of the strategy for the prevention of VAP. The teeth should be brushed every 12 hours with a 1.5 percent peroxide solution and the mouth can be swabbed with an oral sponge containing 1.5 percent peroxide. Every 8 hours, a rinse of .12 percent chlorhexidine gluconate can be applied and then removed by suction. These simple measures can greatly reduce the number of potentially-harmful bacteria located in the oral cavity. Remember to keep the lips moist with a water-based lip moisturizer to keep the lips from cracking, which provides yet another portal for bacteria to reach the patient's system.

- If a patient is on a ventilator for more than 3 days, continuous suctioning of the subglottic secretions that build up in the back of the patient's throat is thought to be helpful. A special endotracheal tube is needed to be able to provide continuous suctioning from a machine, or nursing staff can suction manually every hour or two. Ask about the schedule for suctioning secretions and be sure it happens on time.

- The staff member doing the suctioning should certainly wear gloves on *both* hands, not just on the hand used to manipulate the suction device, because the patient could move or cough and cause the nurse to use the ungloved hand to assist. And the use of protective eyewear and a mask will help prevent any contamination from provider to patient.

- The use of H2 blocker medications to reduce acid and prevent stress ulcers, which are common in intubated patients, is the

usual protocol. Sucralfate is another acid-reducing medication that may be appropriate to use in your situation. The important fact here is that there is a plan of action to prevent the formation of stress ulcers and the potential for GI bleeding, which is a serious situation for ventilated patients.

- Limiting the number of times that the ventilation circuit is "broken" or accessed can help reduce the odds of ventilator-related pneumonia. Inquire if closed or "in-line" suctioning devices would be useful.

- Find out about receiving the pneumococcal vaccine if you are at risk for pneumonia. Anyone who has previously had VAP especially needs the vaccine.

Infection Control at Home

According to the National Association for Home Care, 7.6 million people in the U.S. utilize some form of home health care. Home care workers and family members with no medical training are attending to an increasingly ill patient population. Medical conditions that were serious enough, in the past, to keep people hospitalized are now being treated in the home setting, so it is vital to take proper infection control measures against pathogens in the home environment. A number of factors including complex medical diagnosis in conjunction with IVs, feeding tubes, ventilators, and urinary catheters being used at home, all significantly increase the risk of infection and other complications. People most at risk for infections include newborns, the aged, patients with diabetes, patients with HIV infection or AIDS, people being treated for cancer, patients using any type of catheter, and caregivers themselves (both professional home care personnel and family members).

The following action steps form a rather long list, but the point is to recognize that a person who is recovering from illness, whether it is you or your loved one, is more susceptible to infection than the average person. You want all the surfaces in the house, including people's bodies, to be extra clean and as germ-free as possible.

Action Steps

- I know I'm repeating myself, but the first step in infection control at home is the same as it is in the hospital. Everyone must wash his/her hands regularly and especially before and after any patient contact or after using the bathroom.

- Cleaning supplies, including EPA-registered disinfectants, are needed in the home. Chlorine bleach is an inexpensive, yet effective, disinfectant that can be used for many purposes. Wear gloves when using bleach, and mix one-part bleach to nine parts water. Never mix bleach with any household cleaners containing ammonia since it can start a chemical reaction that causes a gas called chloramine to be produced. Chloramine is highly irritating to the lungs and is potentially toxic.

- Treat all bodily substances as potentially infectious sources, and have both latex exam gloves and rubber "utility" gloves available for use. Clean the rubber utility gloves with the diluted bleach solution mentioned above.

- Patients and caregivers should check with their physicians about any immunizations or vaccines that would help the patient recover, such as those that prevent flu or pneumonia. Professional caregivers should consider being vaccinated for Hepatitis B and having regular TB skin tests.

- In the kitchen, store food carefully by keeping the refrigerator temperature at 40 degrees or less.

- Thaw foods in the refrigerator, and thoroughly cook certain foods—especially meat and eggs, which are notorious for harboring harmful bacteria.

- Use a separate cutting board for meat, and never return cooked meats to the same container or cutting board that raw meat touched.

- Clean your can opener with a disinfectant spray and a scrub brush after each use. A can opener has a history of gnawing open canned foods, and it can keep a little "souvenir" of every food item it has come into contact with. This makes it a special breeding ground for bacteria.

- For the best protection from germs, avoid the use of sponges all together. Disposable paper towels are a safer bet if there is someone in the house at risk of infection.

- Wipe down countertops, and clean the sink regularly with disinfectants.

- Wash your dishes in a dishwasher, or use very hot, soapy water.

- After mopping floors, pour the used mop water into the toilet instead of the kitchen sink.

- Never use your bare hands to wring out a mop. Disinfect the mop in the diluted bleach solution after use. Consider using one of the newer mops with disposable inserts. If you must wring out the mop, wear rubber utility gloves and then clean them in a diluted bleach solution.

- Do not use the kitchen sink for bathing babies or pets.

- In the bathroom, use liquid soap; bar soap, which comes into contact with many, many hands, can harbor bacteria.

- Consider using antibacterial soap for an added measure of infection control if warranted by your medical condition. There is controversy about the efficacy of antibacterial soaps and their ability to increase antibiotic resistance, so don't think of them as a miracle solution to infection. Ask your doctor if you should be using antibacterial soap.

- Change towels and washcloths daily.

- Keep the tub, shower, and bathroom clean with cleanser or the diluted bleach solution.

- Disinfect the toilet by pouring full-strength bleach into the toilet bowl or by putting a bleach tablet into the tank.

- Change toothbrushes every few months and after someone is ill. Toothbrushes can be cleaned by soaking them in hydrogen peroxide or by putting them in the dishwasher. Remember, this is only surface cleaning, not total disinfection.

- Do not share items such as razors, toothbrushes, combs, or hairbrushes.

- Provide disposable cups for drinking water or mouthwash. Do not use mouthwash by putting your mouth on the bottle or by drinking from the cap.

- Wear gloves when doing the laundry if items are visibly soiled with body fluids.

- Dispose of body substances by flushing them down the toilet, and then clean the toilet with bleach.

- Wash contaminated items separately using hot water and bleach. The need for energy conservation has led many people to use only cold or warm water to wash clothes. However, hot water is more effective at eliminating pathogens, which will keep patients with a compromised immune system safe.

- Do not overload the washing machine or the linens will not have sufficient room to agitate in the soapy water, a process that cleans them thoroughly.

- Leave laundry in the dryer until it is completely dry; let clothes that feel even slightly damp dry longer since even a small amount of moisture can encourage the growth of pathogens.

- Change linens weekly or as they become soiled.

- Provide good ventilation to help reduce the number of pathogens in your home. Be aware that modern heating and cooling systems and weather insulation can greatly reduce airflow in your home.

- Realize that pets are another potential host for infections. Immunize your pets, and do not allow patients with weak immune systems to contact bird droppings, fish tank water, or cat litter.

These are general guidelines for improved infection control in the home setting. Consult your physician or home health professional for specific instructions for your infection control needs.

Chapter Four

Medical Errors: A Threat to Public Safety

How to Protect Yourself from Harm

Researchers and the media have compiled mounting evidence to substantiate what many medical patients have known for decades: checking into the hospital is an endeavor that poses a very real risk of injury and/or death. And until now, little has been done to inform patients of the vital part they themselves must play to reduce errors and possibly to save their own life. Because they are so bombarded by decisions, statistics, horror stories from worried relatives, or newspaper reports of the latest hospital lawsuit, they feel completely inept when faced with taking control of their own medical care. Medical patients know intellectually that they must start assuming more responsibility for their outcomes, but because they have no real concept of what that entails, they push the concerns out of their consciousness and assume that they are powerless.

Chapter Four was written to show you that you are anything but helpless in this area. It offers patients and their advocates the skills to assess and identify their particular risk, to evaluate their vulnerabilities, and to employ effective safety strategies. If there is one thing that will keep medical errors on the public's radar screen, it is people tuning into the steady stream of reliable information detailing the considerable number of safety solutions at their disposal, and then speaking up. As many as 98,000 Americans die each year as a result of medical error. These preventable "adverse events" are one of the leading causes of death in the United States—surpassing the number of deaths attributed to motor vehicle accidents (43,000), to breast cancer (42,000), and to AIDS (16,000). Medication errors alone are responsible for one out of every 13 outpatient deaths and one out of every 854 inpatient deaths. Almost two percent of all hospital admissions will include a preventable drug mishap. The statistics might be shocking, but be assured that there are steps you can take to void becoming a victim yourself.

The following 10 boldface headings define separate areas in which medical errors often occur. Understanding the specific errors that plague medical patients, and at what point in the process they tend to happen, is the first step in empowering patients to protect themselves from harm.

Delays in Diagnosis

According to a 2002 report by the Physician's Insurers Association of America, a delay in the diagnosis of breast cancer is the basis for the greatest number of medical malpractice lawsuits in the U.S. Some reports estimate that approximately 40-50 percent of all malpractice claims are initiated because of complications arising from not diagnosing a medical condition correctly and on time. Other conditions at the top of the list of delayed diagnoses include lung cancer, colon cancer, appendicitis, and heart attacks. A timely diagnosis is crucial, and patients risk losing its benefits if the number of tests is inadequate or if their doctor has decided to take a "wait and see" approach when time is of the essence. Other delays occur because there isn't enough follow-up care or the physician or the patient doesn't follow through with consultations with other doctors. There can also be poor communication between doctor and patient or between physician and specialist, an inadequate physical examination and evaluation of symptoms, or the lack of a referral to the right specialist.

Action Steps

- If you sense in any way that you have not been diagnosed properly, don't be shy or intrepid. See another physician immediately.

- Knowing that you've been properly tested is also important. Research which diagnostic tools are available for your symptoms or condition, and understand what information can be gleaned from each type of study. Many cases of breast cancer are missed because physicians do not order breast biopsies so they can thoroughly investigate breast lumps; instead they rely on symptoms and mammograms, which lead to an incorrect diagnosis of benign fibrocystic breast disease. If you don't have Internet access, ask someone who does to do look up your condition and the latest testing options for you, or use a medical research service, in which you pay a nominal fee for a detailed report on all the current information about your condition. Two good places to start are The Health Resource, Inc. at 1-800-949-0090 or www.thehealthresource.com or The California Pacific Medical Center Institute for Health and Healing Planetree Library at 1-415-600-3681 or www.cpmc.org/services/ihh/hhc/research.

- Plan to pay for consults or diagnostic tests yourself if you run into resistance from your insurance company, and fight it later. Don't just give up when the insurance company says no; file a grievance or start an appeal process. In the meantime, don't waste precious time waiting for their answer if you can possibly afford to pay up front.

- If your symptoms intensify or change, alert your physician and immediately report anything new.

- Any ambiguous test results that may suggest an abnormality or which seem unexpected to you should be repeated at a reasonable, predetermined interval. Blood tests that reveal any suspicious results may be repeated immediately to be sure that the original values were not erroneous.

- Don't rely on the doctor to phone you for a follow-up test or scan. Take the initiative to keep track of the time elapsed, and phone to remind them.

- Always trust your intuition. Sometimes you just know when something is wrong.

Errors in Diagnosis

The stories are seemingly endless. A cerebral hemorrhage diagnosed as a migraine, pulmonary embolisms diagnosed as walking pneumonia, patients with stomach cancer being prescribed ulcer medication and released, patients complaining of pain and nausea being told they have the flu and then dying from a ruptured aortic aneurysm. *The Journal of the American College of Chest Physicians, Chest*, published an article in 2001 that examined deaths in ICUs. The researchers found that *one in every five deaths in medical ICU's involved a misdiagnosis*. And in 44 percent of the cases of misdiagnosed patients, a correct diagnosis would have led to different treatments that could have potentially saved the patient's life. Although we all realize that hindsight is 20/20 and some conditions are subtle and will be missed, the medical system continues to miss a significant number of serious and life-threatening conditions. Errors in diagnosis invariably lead to inappropriate and unnecessary tests, ineffective treatment modalities, a decline in the patient's condition and a prolonged recovery.

Action Steps

- The allocation of an appropriate amount of time for a detailed patient evaluation is a prerequisite for a successful diagnosis, so insist on it. When you make the appointment, let the staff know that you are experiencing a problem that may take more than just a few minutes of the doctor's time.

- Don't underestimate the significance of a thorough history, physical exam, and assessment of your symptoms to receive a proper diagnosis. Promising computer technology is being developed to allow doctors to examine a patient and enter information about her symptoms and test results into a database to arrive at the correct diagnosis. Initial results seem highly accurate, but computerized diagnosis is still a long way off, making a thorough, detailed diagnostic process all the more important.

- Take the time to ask that your test results be confirmed by a second reading, especially for x-rays, CT and MRI scans and pathology specimens. Patients can easily be misdiagnosed if their diagnostic information has not been interpreted correctly.

- Familiarize yourself with the simple concept of "differential diagnosis," which is a list of all the disease processes that might be causing the patient's symptoms, in descending order of probability. For instance, a patient arrives at the hospital with three distinct symptoms: fever, vomiting, and a headache. The physician will immediately make a list of the conditions that would explain these symptoms, with the most likely culprit at the top of the list. The doctor will place conditions such as gastroenteritis, viral flu, and infection at the top of the list and a brain tumor way at the bottom. Ask what conditions are being included in your differential diagnosis. Patients who are aware of the "potential" diagnoses can be certain that conditions are systematically removed from the list in a logical manner after the appropriate test has ruled them out.

- In cases of a life-threatening diagnosis, obtain a second, or even third, opinion, which should include giving your history to the new doctor, undergoing a physical exam, and having all previous tests re-evaluated.

Failure to Act on Diagnostic Information

Treatment delays can be caused by inadequate staffing levels, staff members who are poorly trained, the reduced availability of specialists due to cost-cutting measures, emergency room overcrowding, and hospital inefficiency. In other words, you can just fall through the cracks. When doing research for this book, I interviewed Mrs. B, who shared her late husband's story. Mr. B was admitted to a VA hospital with a complaint of kidney stones, and it was determined that a surgical procedure was his best treatment option. As part of his pre-operative testing, Mr. B had blood tests and a chest x-ray, much to the relief of Mrs. B, who worried about her husband's smoking habit. When meeting with the resident to discuss the surgery, Mrs. B pointedly inquired about the results of her husband's chest x-ray. The doctor fumbled through the chart and then told her that the chest x-ray "looked fine." Even though the doctor seemed disorganized and vague, the family did not ask to view the report or think to question any other doctors to confirm the result. The procedure to remove the kidney stones was a great success; however, the radiologist who reviewed Mr. B's chest film had noted a suspicious lesion and recommended immediate follow-up, which was never implemented. It wasn't until months later when Mr. B began coughing up blood that a new x-ray was ordered and compared to the previous film, and the stunned family was informed by an equally shocked medical student that lung cancer had been listed by the radiologist as a possible diagnosis a full nine months earlier. Mr. B lost invaluable time in treating his cancer, and after his untimely death, his family settled a claim with the hospital. Any one of a number of delays can derail a much-needed treatment plan and send you into in a protracted holding pattern—every patient's nightmare scenario.

Action Steps

- Understand what your plan for care is, and be sure to keep yourself updated. That way you will know which tests, treatments, and consultations are pending.

- Ask for a nursing supervisor or a hospital administrator if you feel that your treatment is being delayed because they are short of staff, because of inexperienced staff members, or as a result of just plain inefficiency.

- Let your primary care physician and hospital administrators know if your care was compromised because a specialist was unavailable.

- Don't use hospital emergency rooms unless it's a real emergency. You may be the reason a seriously ill patient is kept waiting.

Tests

The diagnostic tests we depend on to rule out or confirm the presence of illness are inherently prone to inaccuracies. Tests are routinely misinterpreted as a result of inadequate or contaminated samples, miscommunication between healthcare providers, rushed or overworked staff members, and basic human error. Even tests read by computers are not flawless, and can be compromised by the individual programming the machine or by the quality of the sample provided for analysis. Since the information garnered from diagnostic tests guides the decision to operate or provide chemotherapy, radiation, and biopsies, the process can be unforgiving of even the smallest mistakes.

Inadequate or Inappropriate Testing

Inadequate testing can result in potentially serious conditions being missed and crucial treatment being delayed. Tests can certainly be expensive but the price of tests is actually nominal in comparison to the cost of treating lengthy, serious illnesses that could have been prevented if they had been diagnosed in time. It is important to state, however, that not all symptoms initially warrant expensive diagnostic testing. A patient who has a sore knee after jogging doesn't need a MRI scan that afternoon. Traumatic injuries, conditions that become chronic, or a steadily worsening condition are likely to warrant costly scans—but every ache or pain is not an appropriate justification for imaging and will only waste precious healthcare dollars.

Action Steps

- Initiate discussions with your doctors about diagnostic testing, and let them know that you are interested in understanding the rationale for the prescribed course of action.

- Ask the following: Why is the doctor prescribing rest or medication? How long should you wait for improvement? What symptoms could indicate a more serious injury or disease process? If tests are indicated, what are the names of the tests to be ordered? What information is the doctor expecting to gather from each test? Can the information be obtained any other way? Are there any other tests available that the doctor is *not* ordering? Are there any financial factors or insurance restrictions limiting the doctor's ability to order tests?

- You can easily research your symptoms or condition by using the Internet or library books (be sure to check the publishing date—resources need to be up-to-date) and investigate available testing methods. There may be newer testing methods that could be helpful in providing an explanation for your symptoms.

- Research which tests are considered to meet "standard of care" criteria due to their general acceptance by the medical community.

- Contact organizations like the American Heart Association or the Alzheimer's Association to obtain information on recognized testing and treatment standards for a particular disease and for guidance, referrals and support.

Test Results Misread / Misinterpreted

In 1995, a Wisconsin lab pled no-contest to "homicide by reckless conduct" after failing to identify correctly cancerous cells in the PAP smears of two women who later died from metastatic cervical cancer. Lawsuits by the families resulted in huge settlements totaling 9.8 million dollars, after it was revealed that a prompt diagnosis would have afforded the women a 95 percent chance of survival. In 1999, a hospital in Massachusetts contacted 20 men to tell them that their pathology results for prostate cancer were positive. The news came *years* after the men had all been told their results were normal. Scans, x-rays, blood studies, and pathology specimens are all vulnerable to being misread or misinterpreted, sometimes with disastrous consequences.

Action Steps

- Again, patients will be safer if their diagnostic tests are double-checked by a second doctor. Ask about the second doctor's qualifications. Is he a pathologist or radiologist? Does he review scans or x-rays regularly?

- It should be standard operating procedure for all tissue biopsies to be verified by a second pathologist, but you cannot assume that this is the policy of your hospital, so you need to inquire in advance if it will be done. Ask if the pathology lab evaluating your specimen is accredited by the College of American Pathologists and by the Joint Commission.

- Always request a second evaluation of x-rays and scans that confirm or deny malignancies. Some experts recommend that patients have mammograms done at a center where the films will be interpreted by radiologists who devote a minimum of 50 percent of their time to mammography. Ask your mammography center if it is approved by the FDA. Call 1-800-4-Cancer to find a facility in your area.

- Ask if your institution has computer technology available to double-check readings on mammograms or pathology specimens. There is controversy on the benefits of computer analysis for mammography. Recent studies suggest there is no benefit and there may even be an unacceptable number of false positives. The technology is likely to improve, so watch for news on this subject and check with your imaging center.

- Patients can independently seek second opinions of their pathology slides by contacting labs that will provide a second review for a fee. (See Chapter 5)

Test Results Lost or Misplaced

In 1999 the Institute of Medicine reported that missing clinical information is a direct cause of medical error. In 2005 Peter Smith and fellow researchers at the University of Colorado Health Sciences Center found that healthcare providers reported missing clinical information in 13.6 percent of visits. The missing data included test results, medical histories and other treatment information. Missing lab test results were associated with 6.1 percent of all visits. 44 percent of the missing data adversely affected patients and 59.5 percent of the absent test results had the potential to delay care. Lost or mislabeled lab results consume valuable staff time, impair patient safety efforts, and increase healthcare expenditures. In our disorganized and fragmented medical system, wayward lab results are bound to happen; unfortunately, patients continue to pay the price both physically and financially for such inefficiency.

Action Steps

- You can keep your test results safe and accurate by asking that your name and medical record number be stamped on all written orders in the hospital.

- For referrals made in the doctor's office, make sure you understand what test is being ordered and be sure that the requisition is legible.

- At the time of testing, ask when your doctor will be notified of the results. Call the doctor's office to check on your test results if you do not hear from them in a timely manner. No news is not necessarily good news if your results are missing or are filed away before the doctor evaluates them.

- Before you leave your hospital room, ask your nurse to confirm that the lab or x-ray department is in possession of a written or computer order (not just a phone order). Do this before a test is administered, and then question the lab technician yourself to be sure.

- Prevent delays and errors by insisting that your specimen containers be labeled right *before* being used. Never hand a nurse or a patient care assistant a specimen container that doesn't have your name on it! Your sample can easily be mislabeled or mixed up with another patient's, possibly resulting in an erroneous diagnosis or unnecessary treatment. As a safety measure, labs will often refuse to examine unlabeled specimens and may even dispose of them, so if your little vial makes it all the way to the lab without its label, your samples may never be tested. You will wait and wait, and then you'll have to be poked and prodded all over again.

Wrong Test or the Wrong Patient

Even if medical tests were read accurately 100 percent of the time, the study still has to be the appropriate test for a particular set of symptoms, and it must be administered correctly. As absurd as this may seem, gross errors such as ordering the wrong test or administering the right test to the wrong patient continue to plague our healthcare system. A doctor orders a sigmoidoscopy to check for colon cancer, and the test misses a polyp high in the colon that could have been detected and removed immediately if the patient had been given a colonoscopy. A patient undergoes an invasive endoscopy procedure for a complaint of stomach pain, which is eventually attributed to anxiety. The symptoms of irritable bowel syndrome lead to unnecessary ovarian surgery and could have been avoided by ordering a laparoscopic study to look at the organs prior to surgery. Many common ailments, such as gallstones, appendicitis, and heart problems, are misdiagnosed because they all have similar symptoms. Without the proper battery of tests, patients are left without an effective treatment plan.

Action Steps

- Be extremely careful about submitting to tests you were not expecting.

- If your procedure is invasive, conduct a detailed discussion with a physician before signing the consent form. Never sign a consent form if you feel pressured, if you have any doubts, or if you are under the influence of narcotic medications.

- You must know, in full medical terminology, the name of your condition(s) and the names of the tests being ordered by your physician.

- If you are having x-rays and scans, you should know how many views the doctor needs and if your scan will require the injection of any contrast medium or dyes. If contrast is needed, at some point during the scan a technician or doctor will stop the scan to inject dye into the patient or into her catheter. Neglecting to add the contrast medium could necessitate repeating the entire procedure. If one is the least bit claustrophobic, spending another 30 minutes entombed in a MRI machine will be difficult.

- Ask the hospital physician who is ordering the test to notify you of any changes or additions, by telephone if necessary. Let the doctor know that you are not comfortable relying on second-or third-hand information to keep you informed: you want to hear it from your doctor. This will keep you from being wheeled out of your room one day, in a state of bewilderment, listening to the attendant say, "Don't worry; the doctor really did order this test."

- Technicians should always confirm that they have the correct individual, but if they omit this step, you should step up to the plate by confirming your full name, its spelling, your date of birth and the name of the test you are expecting.

No Action or Slow Actions After Test Results are Available

Necessary treatment is often delayed simply because, through a lack of communication, test results weren't reported to the correct person. Sometimes test results are completed but have not been entered into the computer by the lab. They can sit on someone's desk for days. Another frustrating roadblock arises when doctors forget to enter their treatment orders in the patient's chart or computer after they have seen the lab results.

Action Steps

- Ask your nurse or physician to contact the lab directly about pending results that are delaying treatment decisions. Often, information is not entered into the computer immediately due to the demanding workload of laboratory personnel, but the lab staff may have the ability to fax the results to the nurse or to the physician's office to expedite treatment planning.

- Ask your nurse to be sure that the doctor is made aware of important test results and to double-check that any new orders the doctor may have written in light of the new test information are implemented in a timely manner.

Lack of Communication / Miscommunication

PHONE ORDERS

Orders given over the phone for tests, medications or any other prescribed course of action are an obvious source of errors. When investigating the causes of errors, they can regularly be traced back to a miscommunication during phone conversations. Usually, there are no outside witnesses to the conversation (patient and family are not privy to the conversation), and there is the chance that the order won't be written down right away or that the person who is listening is distracted. The person who actually made the error can be impossible to track down, or if he can be found, the "he-said, she-said" argument ensues. Phone miscommunication has been known to result in patients being given medications they are allergic to, in a useless test being ordered for a patient in serious condition, or in an invasive procedure being performed that was completely unnecessary.

The Federal Aviation Administration has long been aware that oral commands can be misinterpreted with deadly consequences. In 1989, an air traffic controller told the pilot of a plane near Malaysia to "descend 2-4-0-0, meaning the pilot needed to descend to 2,400 feet. The pilot interpreted the number "2" as the word "to" and descended to 400 feet. The plane crashed into the side of a mountain and killed all four crew members. In response to such tragic and sometimes unforeseeable miscommunications, the FAA has started a program to allow pilots to communicate with air traffic controllers both verbally and via email messages. Healthcare should be moving in the same direction to protect their patients from preventable errors.

Action Steps

- Whenever possible, try to see that phone orders are avoided altogether. They are an invitation to trouble. Some institutions do not allow phone orders of chemotherapy medications or narcotics because of the potential for deadly errors. Of course, the 3:00 AM calls to physicians for a change in medication are still an integral part of hospital protocol, so vigilance is all the more important.

- Because their level of training ensures that they will understand what is being said, make sure that appropriate staff members, who are usually registered nurses, take phone orders—not secretaries, clerks, or aides. This is technical information about your body being exchanged and it is important that the person taking down the information knows what it means.

- Ask the nurse to take the time to read all orders back to the doctor. If he or she was misheard, the error will be picked up right away. Effective January 1, 2003, the Joint Commission is requiring that the institutions they evaluate "focus attention" on the goal of reading back orders given by phone. Simply repeating back the order does *not* meet Joint Commission standards. The person receiving the order should write down the complete order or enter it into the computer and *then* read it back to the doctor for confirmation. Ask personnel if your hospital is accredited by the Joint Commission, and let them know that you are aware of this recommendation.

- Phone orders should be verified and signed by the physician as soon as they return to the unit.

PROBLEMS WITH HANDWRITTEN AND COMPUTERIZED CHART ENTRIES

The Institute of Medicine reports that illegible medical records have paved the way for thousands of unnecessary deaths. When an entry is unreadable, a busy doctor or nurse might move right along and not take the time to decipher it, which represents another assault on patient's quality of care. It is important to note that even computerized entries (CPOE–Computerized Physician Order Entry), which are easy to read, can contain potentially threatening errors, especially in medications and their dosages, just because of a simple human mistake when the digits were entered.

If you find all this hard to believe, consider this: A third-year pediatric resident at Children's National Medical Center in Washington was quoted in a journal article as saying, "Mistakes are pretty common. I'm used to being called by the pharmacy for ordering the wrong dose." A frightening scenario–but even more chilling when one thinks about what could happen if the pharmacist didn't catch the error. In 1994, *Boston Globe* health columnist, Betsy Lehman, died from a chemotherapy overdose that was four times the correct dose. The error was missed by at least a dozen medical specialists at the Dana-Farber Cancer Institute. This means that there were a number of miniscule windows of opportunity in which this woman's life could have been saved and wasn't. The problem with relying on these "windows" is that if you blink, you miss them. I do realize that problems are bound to occur no matter what safety measures are used because the world is not a perfect place, but the safety net for catching them in the hospital should be more systematic. The practice of finding mistakes should be built into the system, rather than left to happenstance.

Action Steps

- Does the hospital have computer software programs for both physicians and pharmacists in place to catch any obvious errors? Simply entering information about things such as a patient's weight, age, allergies and kidney function tests will catch a slew of potential errors. If not, ask when they plan to invest in this life-saving technology. A demand from informed consumers would help put this tool where it belongs - at the top of the hospital's purchase list.

- In addition to the names of their medications, patients need to know the dosages and have them written down for easy reference.

- In complex treatment plans for diseases such as cancer, there is a predetermined written protocol being utilized. Ask for a copy and familiarize yourself with drug names, dosages and how the medication is to be given and at what intervals.

- Request that your nurses and pharmacists review medication orders written by physicians. Patients with impaired kidney or liver function, known allergies to medications, advanced age, or complicated drug regimens will need staff members to be especially vigilant, since they may be less tolerant of even minor medication errors.

- Ask that a pharmacist consult directly, at your bedside, with your other caregivers since studies have proven that medication errors are reduced when pharmacists are included in daily rounds. The skill of a pharmacist is especially valuable when he or she attends rounds in intensive care units.

DOCTOR/PATIENT COMMUNICATION

With the time allocated for doctor visits on the decline, it's not surprising how easy it is for one party to be misunderstood by the other without realizing it. Since modern medicine allows such limited time for office and hospital visits, patients have to be extremely efficient when communicating with doctors in their allotted time.

Studies have found that the average office visit is about 18 minutes long, including the saying of hello and good-bye and the writing of prescriptions. Within that time, patients have an average of three major concerns to discuss with their doctor. A report in the *Journal of the American Medical Association* found that physicians listen to their patients for an average of 23 seconds before they interrupt them to ask questions. The interruption alone is fine, but the problem is that, after their train of thought is broken off, most patients remain sidetracked and never get around to bringing up their additional concerns. This means that they may leave the office without the majority of their questions even being asked, let alone answered.

Why do physicians tend to interrupt so frequently and so early in the conversation? Their explanation is that patients often deviate from the main issue or give vague descriptions of their symptoms, so doctors feel that they must take control of the situation by interrupting to ask pertinent questions. Their assessment is not necessarily wrong, but as a concerned patient, you need to assert your right to have all your questions dealt with to your satisfaction, no matter how many diversions there are in the conversation.

Action Steps

- You can avoid entering into a game of Twenty Questions if you arrive at your visit completely prepared; you have thought about what to say and how to say it succinctly. Try to allow yourself only two minutes of speaking time; it will force you to get right to the point.

- Don't find yourself in the parking garage after the appointment suddenly remembering some point you were sure you wouldn't forget—but then did. Have your agenda written down in advance, with your most pressing concern at the top of the list.

- List all symptoms, their frequency, and their intensity. Comments like "I feel run down" don't give the doctor much to go on and will set the stage for you to lose your turn at the podium. Specific comments such as "I'm only sleeping four hours a night" or "I feel short of breath whenever I walk up the stairs" provide a much more focused starting point.

- If you feel that your situation warrants allotting the doctor more time than usual, alert the office staff as they are scheduling your appointment so the communication process will not be rushed.

- Don't feel nervous about letting doctors know that you do not understand something or need it explained in a different way.

- You can bring an advocate, a pad and paper, and even a tape recorder to your visit to be sure you don't miss any crucial information. It is difficult to process unfamiliar information and take notes, especially under stress, so ask your advocate to take detailed notes for you. A tape recorder will allow you to listen at a later time to the exact conversation between you and your doctor and may be of assistance to another physician when seeking a second opinion. Of course, be sure you have your doctor's permission.

Caregiver Inter-Communication

Gone are the days of having a single physician who has been treating you for 20 years, making all the decisions concerning your care. Patients now have teams of healthcare professionals managing their treatment. Instead of one captain at the helm of the ship, there are many navigators charting the course, and the patient can only hope that that they are steering the vessel in the same direction. Because each practitioner has his or her own opinions and treatment strategies, it is imperative that all the members of the team have access to each other's orders, thought processes, and rationale for their choices.

Otherwise, decisions will be misinformed, and the way your care is administered will be dangerously fragmented.

This was obvious as I interviewed the daughter of Mrs.C, who relayed the story of her mother's hospitalization for a heart problem and hip pain. Mrs. C's cardiologist decided to treat her irregular heartbeat with a pacemaker, and her orthopedic surgeon recommended hip replacement surgery. The pacemaker was scheduled to be inserted on a Wednesday, and the cardiologist gave the operating room the green light to place Mrs. C on the OR schedule for her hip replacement two days later. As Mrs. C's family scrambled to change their work schedules in order to see their mother through two consecutive surgeries, they expressed their concern to the cardiologist that it might be too overwhelming for an 82 year-old woman to have two surgeries so close together. The doctor assured them that the orthopedist agreed with his assessment, so the family rearranged their schedules, and pre-op blood tests, x-rays, and scans were ordered and completed. Just as Mrs. C was being taken to the OR for her first surgery, the orthopedic surgeon entered the room to tell the family that he had no idea how Mrs. C had gotten on his surgery schedule for Friday, since he had no intention of doing a hip replacement on an elderly woman who had just had a pacemaker implanted. The orthopedist wanted his patient to have time to recuperate from her first surgery and to be sure that the pacemaker was functioning properly before he subjected her to another stressful procedure. Mrs. C's family became acutely aware that the communication between the two was nonexistent while at the same time reassuring their anxious mother that her hip surgery was not being rescheduled due to any problems or complications.

Since communication between consulting members of the team can be limited to reading each other's entries in the medical record, not reading the notes of other providers carefully can cause real problems: unnecessary testing, the repetition of tests, needed tests not being ordered, and medication interactions that create complications. In this day and age of complex treatment, the development of a team approach was meant to benefit patients, but these benefits are negated if the system of communication is broken down.

Action Steps

- Quite simply, you need to request that your providers read each other's entries in the medical record. It may seem unbelievable that you actually have to ask people to do this, but it is often necessary.

- Verify that the individuals involved in your care have conferred with each other and that everyone's input has been considered when implementing the treatment plan.

- Keep a notepad and pen with you at all times so you can make notes about your daily plan for care, and ask each provider if the new tests or medications he is ordering will interfere with or compromise your current treatment plan in any way.

Staff

OVERWORKED, UNDERSTAFFED, OR INADEQUATELY TRAINED

The fact that there are fewer hospital staff members now caring for patients who are more seriously ill has created a work environment that operates, around-the-clock, in overdrive mode. The end result is that the numbers of patient injuries, hospital-acquired infections, and medications dispensed late or missed entirely continue to climb because healthcare providers are forced to struggle with oppressive workloads. Workers simply don't have enough time to pay attention to all the endless details, to recognize every problem before it occurs, or to monitor carefully patients' progress at every juncture during treatment. A nurse who can barely complete her basic duties is not going to have time to educate, comfort, or act as an advocate for her patients.

An additional problem is the practice of replacing highly trained staff members with lesser-trained individuals such as nurse's aides and patient care assistants. A Harvard School of Public Health report in May 2002 confirms what nurses have long pointed out - patients who are cared for by registered nurses have shorter, more problem-free hospital stays. Patient care delivered by RNs has been definitively linked to reduced rates of urinary tract infections, gastrointestinal bleeding, pneumonia, shock, cardiac arrests, and sepsis (infection). The U.S. Department of Health and Human Services issued its final report on nurse staffing and specific patient outcomes and noted that more RNs per shift led to a 3 to12 percent reduction in the measured complication rates.

There is a reason for this. The rigorous training registered nurses receive gives them the knowledge and the resources to facilitate patient recovery and the ability to recognize complications in their earliest stages, when intervention has the greatest chance of success. Unfortunately, aggressive cost containment measures by healthcare institutions have led to a reduction in licensed RNs and more duties being delegated to unlicensed personnel, who are paid significantly less. The trend toward using unlicensed assistive personnel, or UAPs, is especially worrisome, since they can be as young as 18 years old and the recipients of a mere 40-80 hours of instruction. Compounding the problem is that it is left to individual state laws and the discretion of the institution to determine the scope of the duties of assistive personnel; it is not the specific needs of the patient population. Sometimes understaffing doesn't just mean there aren't enough people; it means there aren't enough *qualified* people.

Action Steps

- If you or your advocate sense that the staff is struggling with an unrealistic patient load, you need to initiate tactful discussions with your nurses. The idea is to move the focus, in a non-blaming way, to your concern about your health and not the staff's fallibility. You can do this by an initial expression of regard for their welfare—"It looks as if you're extremely busy"—then gently lead into your own concerns about the safety of your care. For instance, "I'm worried about mistakes being made if people here are too overextended." Keep the remarks about staff general. It is not in your best interest to make anyone feel attacked; you're all in this together, and no one wants mistakes to be made. I myself was surprised at the number of times that nurses and even residents admitted that they were susceptible to making mistakes because of how exhausted they were. Clearly, working long shifts with inadequate staffing levels was not their idea. Remember that they are professionals who value patient safety; appeal to the best in them.

I am dwelling longer on this point because it hits close to home. When my daughter first started receiving chemotherapy, she developed a fever and was admitted to the hospital for IV antibiotic therapy. The antibiotic vancomycin was to be used to protect her from infection since her white blood count was dangerously low. An exhausted resident repeatedly told me that she was writing an order for "vincristine," which was one of Kate's chemotherapy drugs, instead of the antibiotic vancomycin. Before she could even comprehend her mistake, I had to correct her several times. Finally, she confessed that she had been up all night and was having trouble with names. She tried to assure me by saying, "Don't worry. Even if I did order the chemotherapy in error, the pharmacist would catch it." Somehow I did not find this comforting. I shuddered to think what would happen to my daughter's immune system if she were mistakenly given a chemotherapy drug when her blood counts were already dangerously low, and I didn't like the odds of depending on equally overworked pharmacists to be the last safety checkpoint for my beloved daughter.

- Notify the charge nurse, the chief resident, the attending physician, and the hospital administrator if staffing levels seem inadequate. Be suspicious if your medications are late, you don't see your nurse for hours on end, no one responds when you press the call button, or the staff appears to be running ragged. Our highly competitive medical system makes administrators dependent on satisfied customers continuing to seek care at their institutions, so let them know you will go elsewhere if you lack confidence in their ability to staff their hospital.

- Know that UAPs have many titles, including Patient Care Assistants (PCA), Patient Care Technicians and Nursing Aides. Ask what they are called at your hospital.

- Communicate your awareness of the dangers of inadequate staffing, and pass on any harrowing personal experiences to your employer and your insurance company. They're more interested in this issue than you would think because they are the ones who, ultimately, foot the bill for unnecessary complications. If you doubt that employers are serious about this issue, you should know that a national association of Fortune 500 CEOs founded The Leapfrog Group. The group is a coalition of more than 100 public and private organizations that are using their collective purchasing power to alert the healthcare industry that they intend to steer their business to insurance companies and hospitals that meet established safety goals, with staffing being one of their concerns. Visit their website at www.leapfroggroup.org and ask your hospital if they participate in and comply with the goals of the Leapfrog Group.

- Legislators are beginning to realize that they must assume greater responsibility for healthcare safety, so contact their offices and let them know that you are counting on them. Composing a letter or making a personal phone call proves to legislators that you are willing to put precious time and effort into

voicing your opinion; this carries a lot more weight than [
ing a petition or sending an email. California has implemented
AB 394–The Safe Staffing Law–which sets minimum nurse-
to-patient ratios in acute care hospitals. Many other states will
be considering similar legislation, so watch for the opportunity
to support this vital patient safety initiative.

- Make a formal complaint to your State Hospital Licensing
  Board about situations that may have compromised your safety
  (See Chapter 6).

- It's not as if UAPs can or should be banished from caring for
  you altogether, but you can make certain that their duties are
  commensurate with their level of training. Expect UAPs to
  perform certain tasks: taking vital signs, answering call lights,
  assisting with bathing and bathroom needs, and changing
  linens.

- As soon as you are settled into your room, ask to speak to the
  charge nurse so you can inquire about the hospital's policy on
  UAPs and clarify the duties you can expect assistive personnel
  to perform.

- Communicate your expectations to the charge nurse and to
  your physician that you want your more complex medical needs,
  including medication dispensing, dressing changes, and catheter care, are to be managed by a registered nurse. If you feel
  that inexperienced assistive personnel are taking on duties they
  are not equipped to handle, phone the hospital administrator's
  office and ask them to evaluate the situation. It lends you a certain credibility to let them know that you are familiar with the
  Harvard report correlating the number of RNs to safer medical
  care for patients.

RELIANCE ON MEMORY

Because of the hectic pace of the modern day hospital, staff members may resort to relying on their memories as a timesaving strategy. Instead of checking and double-checking the computer, the medical record, or the flow sheet, they try to recollect details on dietary restrictions, medication doses, and allergy identification. This is a flawed and dangerous practice, especially when you consider the deteriorating effect of stress and fatigue on human memory.

Action Steps

- Tell your nurses that you would feel more comfortable if they carried updated copies of your "flow sheet" or a copy of the physician's orders with them while providing your care (many nurses do this routinely). Besides general orders by the physician, flow sheets include information about activity levels, diet, tests, and medications. All medications are listed by name, and detailed instructions are given regarding the route of administration and the times medication are administered.

- Strive to be a true partner in your care by requesting your own copy of the daily flow sheet or computerized physician's orders to keep at your bedside to pencil in notes to help you understand the orders.

- Check off each order on the flow sheet as it is completed so your care is never compromised by simple forgetfulness.

Surgical Mishaps

WRONG SITE, WRONG PATIENT OR
WRONG PROCEDURE SURGERY

One of the most famous cases of wrong-site surgery involved Willie King of Tampa, Florida. The unfortunate Mr. King entered the hospital to have his gangrenous right foot amputated, but an egregious series of errors resulted in the removal of his left foot instead. Of course, afterwards, the gangrenous right foot still needed to be amputated, which left Mr. King without feet at all and virtually no prospect of ever walking again.

USA Today reported in April, 2006 that wrong site surgery is increasing, despite all efforts to eliminate this medical error. Last year, healthcare organizations reported 84 incidents of wrong site surgery or wrong patient surgery to the Joint Commission. A few states mandate such reporting of errors, but a large majority don't, and errors occurring at these hospitals may never be made public. Dr. Dennis O'Leary, the president of the Joint Commission is quoted in *USA Today* in 2006 as saying "I can assure you that this is just the tip of the iceberg. Some hospitals are reporting everything and some hospitals don't report anything at all."

There is no one definitive source that provides the public with the total number of wrong-site surgeries performed in the U.S. each year, because we don't have a national, mandatory reporting system for such errors. Imagine if each airline quietly investigated its own near-misses, emergency landings and crashes because we didn't have the FAA to arrive at the scene within hours, investigate incidents and mandate quality-control measures. Of course, some of these surgeries were not carried through to their conclusion because the mistakes were caught while the patients were still opened up, so they were, in effect, wrong-site "almost" surgeries.

Another terrifying story is that of Carl Graham of Tallahassee, Florida, who went into the OR for surgery on one lung and came out with large incisions on both sides of his torso. Obviously, the error was caught on-site because the surgeon closed the first incision and then completed the surgery on the correct lung. "Almost" errors are even more difficult to track down; patients might either overlook the mistake and thus never mention it, or settle quickly with the hospital or doctor for a nominal sum of money, which may not require the doctor to report the settlement to medical boards.

According to the National Patient Safety Foundation, one in four orthopedic surgeons, at some point in their career, will operate on the wrong site. It is a relatively rare occurrence, yet it is completely indefensible because it is 100 percent preventable. It is the result of a failure of the entire system and usually involves a series of errors by several individuals. A clerical error lists the wrong body part on a form, x-rays are not reviewed in advance, x-rays are mounted backwards on a view box, or a nurse mistakenly drapes the wrong side of the body.

A patient interviewed for this book, Mr. JWB, gave an account of his brush with a wrong site surgery scare. Mr. JWB was slightly sedated while waiting in a pre-op area prior to surgery for a total hip replacement on his right side. In walks a nurse and announces that she needs to confirm the surgical location and announces that Mr. JWB is having a total hip replacement on his left side. Mr. JWB, a little woozy from his sedative, thinks the nurse is having a little fun at his expense, and laughingly tells her, "Actually, I think I'll have a hip replacement on the right side." The nurse looks at him sternly and says that she doesn't think it's very funny to try to confuse her about the surgical site. Mr. JWB now realizes that this is no joke; the paper in the nurse's hand actually states that the hip replacement is on his left side instead of his right. After emphatic protests by Mr. JWB, the surgeon was consulted and the mistake corrected before any real harm was done.

In 1998, in response to this growing phenomenon, the American Academy of Orthopedic Surgeons (AAOS) initiated a "sign your site" campaign that encouraged surgeons to initial the surgical sites in advance right on patients' bodies to make absolutely sure that they were operating on the right place. In an attempt to appeal directly to healthcare facilities, in July 2003 the Joint Commission adopted a "universal protocol" to prevent wrong site surgeries. This protocol has four components: 1. A pre-op verification process that includes a review of all notes, confirms that all studies and test results are present and reviewed and checks the intended patient, the correct procedure and the right surgical site. 2. The surgical site is marked by the surgeon. 3. A "time-out" is taken by the team as a last opportunity to confirm the patient, procedure and the site. 4. The above three steps are also applied to non-operating room settings, such as procedures done at the bedside or in a treatment room.

Unfortunately, even with the above mentioned universal protocol, wrong site surgeries continue to occur. In June, 2006 a patient in the Veterans Affairs Medical Center in Los Angeles erroneously had a healthy testicle removed, leaving him with one atrophied and painful testicle. All the more distressing is that the Veterans Administration is looked to as one of the pioneers in wrong site surgery prevention. Even with specific systems in place, a cascade of errors and omissions led to the disastrous outcome. The consent form listed the wrong testicle as the one to be removed, and both the patient and the doctor signed it. I can't imagine how the surgeon signed it, but the patient signed it *without reading it and without wearing his glasses.* The patient recalls pointing out the surgical site, but it was not marked with a pen. Again, the lesson here is crystal clear: it is not sufficient to point to a body part and then assume that everything will run smoothly after you are asleep. DO NOT allow yourself to be put under without the surgical site being marked. Finally, the medical record states that a time-out was called, but the information being confirmed was incorrect. Even when there is a "system" in place to protect you, patients cannot be complacent about being vigilant and following through by checking every detail.

Action Steps

- Insist that your surgeon signs the operative site in marking pen. The Veterans Administration directive on wrong-site surgery dictates that patients should not mark a non-operative site in any way. For example, if you are having surgery on your right knee, they do not recommend marking the left knee with the word "No" or "Other Knee." Depending on what you choose to write on the non-operative knee, it is felt that a variety of marks could actually lead to more confusion. Certainly, ambiguous marks such as an "X" should never be used. One of the solutions to this problem is for *all* surgeons to initial *every* surgical site and never start a procedure unless they see their own initials.

- Let the staff know that you will not be signing the consent form until your surgical site is marked. Remind them of the directive by the Joint Commission.

- Be sure to ask if your medical record and any imaging studies have been delivered to the operating room so they are readily available at the start of surgery.

- Confirm the surgical site with the OR nurse and the anesthesiologist.

- Having surgery at a Joint Commission-accredited facility will at least ensure that the hospital is expected to have a policy for marking surgical sites, will be questioned about their policies for avoiding wrong-site surgery, and that any deficiencies have potentially been discovered and eliminated.

LACERATIONS OR EXCESSIVE BLEEDING

Lacerations and perforations are unintentional (and sometimes undetected) cuts, nicks, tears, or other entries into blood vessels or organs. Lacerations can be small, resulting in a slow leakage of blood or fluid that may not be detected for hours or even days, or they can be big enough to sever large vessels completely and lead to a life-threatening loss of blood. Perforations into organs such as the bowel with scalpel blades or other instruments can cause temporary trauma or permanent damage. If the contents of the bowel somehow spill into the abdominal cavity, it greatly increases the chance of infection. Large bowel perforations can be serious; they may necessitate removal of the damaged portion of the intestine and the reliance on a colostomy procedure during the recuperation phase. The wounds themselves aren't necessarily dangerous; it's what they lead to that's the problem because they can create the need for additional surgery to correct the injury, provide places for bacteria to grow, trigger excessive bleeding that can lead to shock, and cause significant delays in recovery.

Often patients don't even realize that a laceration or perforation has occurred during their procedure; they never fully understand why they're in so much pain, why they've developed an infection, require additional surgery, or have a protracted recuperation period. The new approach to reducing medical errors calls for open, honest discussions about mishaps, and direct inquiries from patients and their advocates are an effective starting point.

Action Steps

- Have an advocate who will be present at the conclusion of your procedure to speak with the surgeon to discuss the details of the surgery while they are fresh in the doctor's mind.

- Advocates can help determine if there were any surgical complications by asking focused questions such as "Was there any excessive bleeding during the procedure?" and "Did you have to perform any additional procedures during the surgery due to unforeseen complications?"

- If you're experiencing problems in recovery and you suspect this type of error, the key is asking your doctor point-blank. Remember, a vague question will invite only a vague answer, so knowing the correct terminology is helpful. Ask, "Were there any surgical mishaps? Were there any lacerations or perforations during my procedure?" Of course, the doctor could be less than truthful, but when faced with a direct question, this is both unlikely and unethical.

- Be sure that your surgeon is aware of any blood-thinning medications you're taking, which makes any cuts more threatening, and ask how far in advance of the surgery you should stop using them. Be extra vigilant that blood-thinning medications are not given in error before a surgical procedure.

INSTRUMENTS OR SUPPLIES LEFT IN PATIENTS

In January 2003, the results of the largest study of surgical tools being left inside patients revealed that at least 1,500 people each year are victimized by this error. In June 2001, the city of San Francisco settled a lawsuit in which two objects were left in the body of a woman after two separate surgical procedures. During the first operation, a blue surgical towel was left in the patient's abdomen, and no one stumbled across it until six months later, by which time it had eroded the wall of her large intestine. The next surgery, whose express purpose was to remove the misplaced towel, included a temporary colostomy procedure. Three months later during the surgery to reverse the colostomy, part of the rubberized tubing used as a drain for the colostomy bag was left in the patient's abdomen. Such surgical mishaps are relatively rare, but in this poor woman's case, lightning struck twice.

Action Steps

- Inform yourself of the strict protocols your hospital has in place to count instruments before a surgical site is closed, and expect them to adhere to them. The responsibility of counting instruments is usually assigned to a specific operating room nurse. Unfortunately, the 2003 study showed that in two-thirds of the surgeries that resulted in retained surgical instruments, an instrument count was performed both before and after the procedure, so it is not a definitive solution to the problem. Certainly, instrument counting is far from perfect, but we cannot discount its value.

- If your surgery is scheduled in advance, you can call the hospital and ask to speak to the operating room nurse supervisor about the safeguards your hospital has in place to prevent this type of error. Even when a surgery is unplanned, you can speak to your OR nurse directly as you enter the operating area.

- Be aware that obese patients have a higher incidence of surgical tools being left in their bodies. If this applies to you, taking an x-ray before the wound is closed may be useful in double-checking that all instruments are accounted for.

- Patient's undergoing emergency surgery and those who experience an unexpected change in surgical procedure have a higher incidence of retained surgical instruments, so any unusual post-surgical pain or complications should be looked at with extra care in these individuals.

- If you plan to be sedated ahead of time, ask your pre-operative nurse to speak to the operating room nurse for you. Informed patients who inquire about protocols to prevent leaving supplies in patient's bodies will at least guarantee that the subject is on the minds of the surgical team while they are working and hopefully raise the performance bar for all of them.

- Be aware that there is new technology to help locate retained sponges in surgical sites. Sponges to be used during surgery are tagged with a radiofrequency identification chip (RFID) and then, at the end of the surgery, a handheld wand is passed over the patient to see if it detects a radiofrequency signal. This is a new technique, but in early testing it seems to be effective. It would certainly be helpful in the high-risk situations mentioned above. Ask your surgeon if "tagged" sponges are available in your hospital.

SURGICAL FIRES AND OTHER SOURCES OF PATIENT BURNS

The idea of a fire breaking out in the OR does not even occur to most people, so you would be surprised to learn that fire is an ever-present risk in operating rooms. There are approximately one hundred operating room fires reported each year, but this is only the number of incidents that are disclosed – the number is likely higher since reporting is voluntary in almost every state in the country. Three elements often referred to as the "fire triangle" – heat, fuel and oxygen – come together and start a sudden and intense flash fire. Heat sources in the OR include overhead lights, electrosurgical or electocautery tissue-cutting devices (sometimes referred to as a Bovie), lasers, drills and defibrillators. A fuel source is literally anything that can burn including surgical drapes, gowns, linens, skin prepping agents such as ether, acetone or alcohol, gauze, sponges, tape, ointments, breathing masks and hair. The oxidizer is oxygen or nitrous oxide gas, which creates on oxygen enriched environment and can leak into the air from the patients mask or the nasal area. Even though the elements of the fire triangle are present in the OR *every* time surgery is performed, it is 100% preventable. Imagine your reaction at being told that your sinus surgery was a great success, but the burns on your face, which weren't there when you were wheeled in, will take months to heal and require additional corrective surgery.

Fires and burns that occur outside the OR can be caused by the use of caustic chemicals, MRI scans, the improper use of electricity and microwave ovens and by patients themselves (from trying to sneak a cigarette, for example).

Action Steps

- Ask the surgeon if a cautery unit will be used in your surgery, and verify that precautions are in place to prevent a fire. Ask your surgeon if he and his staff know how to put out an operating room fire.

- Draping the head may present a higher risk due to oxygen pooling under the drapes so ask if your head needs to be covered during head or neck surgery.

- The skin prep used to clean your skin must be completely dry in order to minimize the risk of a fire. Ask the staff to be sure that they give the prep enough time to dissipate.

- Ask if you can breathe room air or no more than 30% oxygen, since 100% oxygen carries a greater risk of igniting a fire.

- Facial hair should be covered in water soluble jelly. Do not shave any skin in the surgical field right before surgery as you can cause cuts in the skin which may allow bacteria into your body.

- Know that gauze and sponges can be kept moist in the operating room to reduce flammability.

- Ask your surgeon if a surgical fire has ever occurred at this hospital or happened to him or her personally. Do staff members receive training on prevention and management of surgical fires? The surgeon may be surprised that you're even aware of this danger—but he or she will be that much more cautious when working on you.

- Check the website www.surgicalfire.org for valuable information and helpful links.

- You must abide by the strict non-smoking regulations at your health care institution—for your own safety and the safety of other patients. If you are worried about nicotine withdrawal symptoms, ask your doctor if using a nicotine patch, chewing gum, or nasal spray is appropriate during hospitalization.

- Be certain that any chemical solutions applied to your skin are prepped and applied by experienced personnel. Insist on a small test area first to determine any ill effects.

- Be aware that the VA National Center for Patient Safety has reported on patients sustaining burns during MRI scans from looped ECG leads, pulse oximeter cables touching the skin, or from the ignition of special cuffs or sleeves that remain in contact with patients during the scan. These devices contain electrically conductive materials and have the ability to hold heat. Very rarely, tattoos or permanent eyeliners containing iron oxide have also heated and caused minor burns. Realize that sedated patients will be at a greater risk for burns since they will not feel discomfort. Ask the technician to double-check all wires, leads, cables and cuffs. If possible, don't have wires or cables cross over each other, and don't let them touch the patient unless absolutely necessary. Always check underneath blankets and hospital gowns for any potentially conductive wires or cables that may have been missed.

ANESTHESIA

Complications from anesthesia range from mild to life threatening. Nausea is a common side effect, but it rarely causes serious problems. At the other end of the spectrum is the case of then 39-year-old Denise DeSoto. In 1993, Mrs. DeSoto was in a car accident and had surgery on her hand at a California university medical center. A week later, circulation in her hand was severely compromised; consequently, another surgical procedure had to be performed. Thirty minutes after her second hand surgery, Denise DeSoto suffered a cardiac arrest and extensive brain damage from a lack of oxygen. The culprit? A breathing tube clogged with mucus, which was monitored by a medical resident with a mere five months of anesthesia experience. The lawyer for the DeSoto family stated that it took more than three years of litigation before the hospital's attorneys would admit that the resident had been the acting anesthesiologist. In 1998, Judge C. Robert Jameson awarded the family almost 19 million dollars and found that the university had "stonewalled from the get-go" and that the hospital tried to prevent the court from learning the truth about the cause of Mrs. DeSoto's brain damage through "intentional, despicable, unprofessional" conduct.

The DeSoto family thought that Denise's biggest problem was her injured finger. What they didn't understand is that when she walked through those hospital doors, she had her initial problem of a lacerated finger, which we'll call Problem A. But then came along Problem B—a loss of oxygen to her brain from a completely preventable complication. Problem B sometimes makes Problem A look like a walk in the park.

Action Steps

- Insist on meeting with your anesthesiologist prior to surgery to review your health history, allergies, medications and any other pertinent information.

- The tragic story of Denise DeSoto proves that an experienced anesthesiologist is a necessity, so ask if the one monitoring you while you're unconscious is board certified in anesthesiology. Even if a resident is performing your anesthesia, a board-certified anesthesiologist should be carefully monitoring the entire surgery in person.

- It is safer for infants and very young children to be sedated by a pediatric anesthesiologist, so if your child is having surgery, ask if the hospital has them on staff.

- Ask if any students or residents will be participating in the anesthesia process in any capacity whatsoever, so you will know ahead of time what role less experienced personnel will have in your surgery.

- Determine in advance how post-operative issues like nausea, vomiting, or a headache will be handled and ask if the anesthesiologist will be the one managing your post-op needs. If not, whom should the nurses contact if you have side-effects related to your anesthesia?

Systems or Procedure Errors

Systems errors are mistakes that occur over and over simply because the way that procedures and protocols are set up is inherently faulty. They are flaws in the organization of healthcare delivery and have already been identified as contributing factors in the epidemic of medical errors. Not only is the system faulty, but it is not designed to catch its own faults. Consequently, obvious errors are allowed to happen over and over again, and unfortunately have the unmitigated power to repeatedly victimize thousands of patients. The only way to prevent some of these mistakes from happening on an ongoing basis is to identify and correct the original flaw in the system.

A simple metaphor here is the operating systems in computers. Anyone experienced with computers knows that if there is a problem in the operating system, the same error will occur at every application until someone catches it and then corrects the original problem.

Mrs. DC told me about an incident regarding her husband that illustrates how often poor outcomes go unchecked in our current system. Mr. DC had been hospitalized for a knee operation and was given a medication to help him sleep. Unfortunately, Mr. DC had a bad reaction to the drug and suffered from anxiety and mild hallucinations. The family discussed the reaction with the nurses and the doctor, and it was agreed that the sleeping medication was the culprit. Mr. DC's family just assumed that the drug would be discontinued, but never confirmed this fact with the staff. Mr. DC suffered through another night of hallucinations because the order to stop the medication had never been entered into the computer, and the pharmacist sent up another dose of the sleeping pill, which the evening nurse administered. Having a set hospital protocol in place for reporting, documenting, and discontinuing medications that cause dangerous side effects would prevent such adverse drug reactions from reaching the same patient twice. As another layer of protection, patients need to write down changes and confirm that they are implemented.

Some of the most persistent systems errors occur because of simple things such as poor handwriting, which causes endless miscommunication. Healthcare institutions not only tolerate poor handwriting, they don't install enough safeguards in their systems to eradicate it. By not addressing this simple problem at its source, hospitals allow the mistakes that arise from illegible notes to permeate and plague their systems.

LACK OF STANDARDIZATION IN HOSPITAL PROTOCOLS AND SYSTEMS

Standardization is the process by which irregularities and "personal styles" are removed from the way that staff is allowed to operate medical devices. There is no room for creativity or innovation when doing things like programming IV pumps. These highly technical machines are designed to be operated with a certain protocol, or they cannot be counted on to function as they should, and healthcare institutions simply do not put enough effort into implementing policies that would standardize their systems.

Large institutions are notorious for dragging their feet when it comes to making system-wide changes. Institutional administrators continuously debate factors such as cost, additional employee training, and increased paperwork, and often completely miss the big picture: lives will be saved, suffering will be avoided, and ultimately, these safety measures will lower costs by reducing the expenditures on treating people victimized by errors.

Action Steps

- Let your healthcare institutions know that you expect them to consider state-of-the-art safety measures like computerized entry, bar coding, and handheld computers a necessary investment.

- Check to see if the institution you are in has procedures in place that actually make it difficult for staff members to make errors. Just recently, my bank instituted a simple new step that reminded me how easy it would be for hospitals to do the same.

After I enter the amount of my deposit, the machine asks me if this is correct, and I have to hit a button to confirm the deposit. These steps are called "forcing functions" because they require us to stop, think, and then confirm that we really did ask for what we think we asked for. We need more of these in healthcare. Institutions should immediately implement the following specific policies:

1. Utilize computers to enter electronic prescription orders. Say good-bye to illegible handwriting and hello to software programs that do extraordinary things like identifying drug interactions and recognizing dosages that are out of range.

2. Invest in technology (such as handheld computers) containing medical reference information for nurses and physicians. An accurate, state-of-the-art database can alert healthcare providers to drug interactions, errors, and misdiagnoses.

3. Include a pharmacist on rounds to assist physicians in choosing the correct medications and dosages. Pharmacists could function as another safeguard for patients by working directly with physicians, accessing detailed patient information via the computer, and double-checking for allergies and drug interactions.

4. Standardize medical equipment and standardize procedures by having providers stop at predetermined points in patient care duties to fill in checklists and initial them to signify that all appropriate precautions have been followed. To reduce medication errors, hospitals need to institute a program in which personnel scan the bar code on medication vials and then scan a bar code on the patient's wristband to be sure they coincide.

5. Have a mandatory review policy for all narcotic orders and all dosages of pediatric medications.

CONCENTRATED DRUGS NOT DILUTED PROPERLY AND ERRORS IN DOSAGE STRENGTH

Concentrated drugs are potent forms of medications that are meant to be diluted and dispersed in different strengths. They are rarely administered in their original strength, yet that is the condition in which they are packaged and stored. In the recent past, patient deaths have been attributed to the practice of keeping highly concentrated drugs on the medical unit or, worse yet, right at the patient's bedside. Ideally, these bottles should have been kept exclusively in the pharmacy, but for the sake of convenience, they were sometimes stored on patient floors.

Concentrated drugs have been implicated in fatal overdoses either by being given full strength or by not being diluted correctly before being administered to patients. Concentrated potassium chloride (KCl) is a well known example of a drug with a history of being given to patients in undiluted form and has led to cardiac arrest and death. The Joint Commission issued a sentinel event alert and a simple change in the system of storing KCl has virtually eliminated this error.

In September of 2006, the nation witnessed the tragedy of six premature infants erroneously given adult doses of the blood thinner heparin. The adult dose is 1,000 times the prescribed amount of heparin for newborns. As packaged, the adult dose and the pediatric dose of heparin look very similar. A pharmacy technician stocked the adult dose of heparin into a medication-delivery cabinet for the NICU, which was then dispensed by the nurses on duty. Three of the babies died from the overdose and, in an unbelievable twist in the story, two babies were overdosed with heparin *five years* earlier in *the same hospital.*

Action Steps

- Ask if concentrated drugs needed for emergency use are stored only in the pharmacy or on a crash cart.

- Check to see if any of your medications need to be diluted before being given.

- Familiarize yourself with the drugs that pose the greatest risk for patients, and ask if they will be used in your treatment: potassium chloride (KCl), potassium phosphate, anticoagulants such as heparin, insulin, opiates and other narcotics, and concentrated sodium chloride (NaCl).

- If any of the above drugs are being used in your treatment plan, ask before every dose is administered if it is the correct concentration. Be especially vigilant about children, as they are less likely to be able to endure a drug overdose.

- Be aware that hospitals accredited by the Joint Commission are required to have a policy in place for storing concentrated drugs. Because it is human nature to revert back to bad habits when not under scrutiny, realize that there is always the possibility that concentrated drugs could be stored in places that endanger patients, even if the hospital has a policy against this practice.

- Always ask the staff member who is administering any medication to stop and check the dose and the concentration.

BAR CODING

Bar coding is simple, cost-effective technology developed years ago that has yet to be used widely in the healthcare system. Major patient safety organizations such as the Institute of Medicine, the National Patient Safety Foundation, and the Center for Disease Control have all reported that bar coding is under utilized as a life saving measure in medical applications. The Food and Drug Administration, under pressure from advocacy groups, has mandated bar coding on the labels of thousands of drugs and biological products. The bar codes will be required on most prescription drugs and on all blood products. Of course, on the other end, there needs to be technology in place in the hospital or pharmacy to scan the barcode to ensure the right drug is going to the right patient.

Bar coding that can be scanned by pharmacists can be placed on medication labels right at the manufacturing plant. In addition, it can be added to the wristbands of patients for scanning prior to administering medications or performing tests and applied to medical records to prevent loss or mix-ups. In an era of rapidly rising healthcare expenditures, the main resistance to bar coding by drug companies and healthcare institutions is the cost. Bar coding has been used in retail stores for 30 years now. Grocery stores have managed to bar code everything from hamburger to dish soap without going bankrupt. We're lucky that stewed tomatoes will never be mistaken for refried beans, but in a hospital, Zantac could be confused with Xanax.

Action Steps

- Determine if bar coding technology is available at your institution, and ask that it be used in your care whenever possible.

- Check the information on your wristband for accuracy, and wear your wristband at all times. You will be safer if your wristband had two patient identifiers on it. No one can be expected to memorize her medical record number, so your full name and your birth date should also be clearly visible on your wristband.

- In lieu of bar-coded information, ask to wear an additional brightly colored wristband to identify any allergies, fall risks, seizures, and so on.

- Let your healthcare institutions, physicians, and your government representatives know that you consider bar coding technology to be an essential safety measure that you would like to see implemented in the hospital setting in the near future.

PLACEMENT OF DECIMALS

The seemingly minor mistake of a misplaced decimal, in the health care setting, can be lethal. If a patient needs .01 mg of a drug but is given .1 mg in error, she has received 10 times what she should be taking. In 1996, a two-month-old child in Texas was administered 0.9 milligrams of digoxin, a heart medication. The appropriate dose was .09 milligrams, one tenth of the dose given. The overdose of digoxin caused the infant's heart to stop beating, and he died 30 minutes later. One would think that this tragic incident would have resulted in a nationwide change in policy regarding decimals so that other families would not lose a child because of a dot on a piece of paper. The reality is that our fragmented medical system has no means to disseminate information about errors to hospitals and that we have no governing entity with the authority to require immediate change and compliance. The "recommendations, not regulations" policy of our healthcare leadership continues to place patients at risk for injury.

Action Steps

- Ask your hospital if they have a policy that requires a leading zero to be used for *all* medication orders. A leading zero is an immediate heads-up that the dose is less than one percent. This is important because many medication errors occur because of the possibility of confusion about concentrations involving one percent. Imagine all the possible mistakes - .01%, 0.10%, 1.0%, 0.001%, etc. All orders without a leading zero should be automatically rejected; staff should be required to reorder the dose after consultation with a physician.

- Know your dose! Are you supposed to receive .01mg of a drug or .1 mg? It can be easy to confuse these dosages, but the second one is *ten times* the amount of the first one.

- Expect all orders to be reviewed at the pharmacy and for questionable orders to be placed in a designated area where they cannot be mistakenly filled until confirmed with a physician.

- See if your orders can be entered via computer, which will eliminate mistakes from illegible handwriting. In addition, software is available that can alert healthcare providers to dosages that might be out of range for your age or weight.

- Remember that it is not that uncommon for computers to be "down" due to maintenance, system updates, or crashes. Total reliance on computers for clarity and accuracy is not a perfect solution; the institution must be committed to demanding legible entries from staff members and using regular checkpoints to confirm accuracy in the event that the computer system is unavailable.

- Ask physicians to use zeroes wisely in their written orders and to double-check all decimal points.

- Have your nurse check for correct decimal placement.

- Know that the pharmacist should not fill your prescriptions unless the doctor has entered information about your age, weight, height, diagnosis, and renal function, since all can affect medication dosages.

- Ask nurses to confirm that the ordered dose matches the information listed on the label before they administer any medication.

MEDICATION ERRORS

The Institute of Medicine report, *To Err Is Human*, acknowledges that "medication-related errors occur frequently in hospitals." A 1993 article published in the medical journal *Lancet* found that medication errors accounted for approximately 7,000 deaths that year alone.

A 1995 study found that almost two percent of hospital patients experience an "adverse drug event," meaning that their medication error resulted in actual bodily harm. In July of 2006, the National Academies released a new report stating that medication errors injure 1.5 million Americans every year. Perhaps the most stunning statistic included in this report is that a hospitalized patient can experience one or more medication errors every day.

The medical research community readily admits, however, that estimates of the number of medication errors are low because of the lack of documentation in medical records and because of underreporting by hospitals. The saddest truth of this is that children are more vulnerable to this type of error than adults, since children are at an increased risk for medication errors. The greatest number of these kinds of mistakes occurs in Pediatric Intensive Care Units. The results of a four-year study, published in 1989, found a medication error rate of one per 6.8 admissions in neonatal and pediatric intensive care units. A 2004 study found an 11.1 percent prescribing error rate in nine pediatric intensive care units evaluated. Safety improvements reduced the number to 7.6 percent – still a significant risk.

PRESCRIBING

Safety experts have determined that one of the major factors in medication errors is inaccurate prescribing. Such errors can occur if the wrong drug has been ordered, if the dose of a drug is inappropriate, if the dose interval is incorrect, if the patient's medical history has not been evaluated thoroughly, if prescribed medications interact with each other in harmful ways, or if the doctor uses abbreviations when writing out the prescription. Patients with impaired hepatic (liver) or renal (kidney) function may require drug dosages that would be different from other patients, a fact that can be overlooked by medical personnel.

The most common factors leading to errors in prescribing medications involve the doctor's ability to utilize his knowledge about drug regimens accurately and to correctly evaluate all the pertinent patient information that may affect drug selection. A study by Kozer, et al published in the October 2002 issue of *Pediatrics* found prescribing errors in 10.1 percent of the charts of children treated in the emergency department. Children treated between the hours of 4 AM and 8 AM, children with serious disease processes, and children seen on the weekends were at an increased risk. A 1997 article in the medical journal *Heart & Lung* revealed that nurses at a Dallas hospital were unable to read one in five medication orders written by the 36 physicians caring for patients on three different wards. Almost 25 percent of the medication orders were incomplete, and 78 percent of the signatures on the orders were unrecognizable. The last thing you want is nurses or pharmacists having to make "educated guesses" about your medications because they cannot figure out which doctor to call for clarification or confirmation.

Action Steps

- You have the ability to institute your own policy, to some degree, simply by asking your caregivers to write clearly in your medical record and on any prescriptions.

- Discuss your drug therapies with your doctors, and keep a list of all the medications ordered, their dosages, and times to be administered, via a copy of the physician's orders.

- Be truthful about all the drugs you have taken, including illicit drugs, herbal remedies, and over-the-counter medications. Be honest about your use of tobacco products and alcohol.

- Ask for a pharmacist to be directly involved in your treatment planning, especially if you have a complex drug regimen. Some hospitals are now utilizing "satellite pharmacies" on specialized units such as oncology floors and intensive care units to provide the expertise of a pharmacist right on site who is familiar with the patients and their drug regimens. Let your hospital know that you believe this would make care safer and more efficient.

- Ask your physicians to avoid the use of abbreviations when writing orders, since many drugs are spelled alike and the use of abbreviations can easily lead to errors.

- Inquire into a hospital policy requiring all handwritten prescriptions to be done in block printing, a far more deliberate and legible form of the written language than handwriting. It would be a solution that is simple, effective - and free. Better yet, see if your hospital is using computerized drug ordering systems.

- Ask to view your record periodically, or ask a family member to verify that the writing is legible.

- See if your hospital has a standard policy for the use of decimal points, preferably one that requires the use of a leading zero.

- Since many medication errors involve patients receiving medications to which they have known allergies, make a big deal about your allergies and discuss them with all hospital personnel who handle your care. Allergies should be noted on your wristband, on the front of your chart, and above your bed.

- Keep a record of the details of all allergic reactions and any prior unpleasant side effects of medications.

- If a certain medication worked well for you in the past, make a note of it so you will be readily able to communicate its name and dosage to hospital staff.

ADMINISTERING MEDICATIONS

Error rates in the preparation and administration of medications have been reported in the literature to be as high as 19 percent. Errors in dispensing medications from the pharmacy can be caused by the multitude of drugs that look alike or have similar sounding names. Hospital personnel who administer medications must have the right patient, the right drug, the right dose, the correct route of adminis-tration, and the right time or interval. When considered individually, each of the duties involves relatively simple actions. But when you combine all of the requirements listed above and factor in conditions like illegible handwriting, staffing shortages, poorly documented allergies, and the inability of elderly or debilitated patients to com-prehend their extensive drug regimens, the process takes on a fright-ening complexity. Even a mix-up of over-the-counter medications can cause a patient great discomfort.

Mrs. H recounted an incident to me in which she asked her nurse for a dose of Maalox to calm her stomach. After checking with a physician, the nurse came into her room with a small, single-dose container of a white liquid. After swallowing the medication, Mrs. H suspected that she had not been given Maalox, so she fished the container out of the garbage to discover that she had just swallowed milk of magnesia. Not a life-threatening situation, but needless to say, Mrs. H's stomach was not going to feel better any time soon.

Action Steps

- Know the names of all medications you take at home, includ-ing generic and brand names. The drug Lasix, for instance, is also known as furosemide, and Coumadin is also called warfa-rin. Have all your medications (both names), the dosages, and the time of day that they are taken, written down and easily accessible.

- What do your medications look like? What is the size, color and marking on the pills? You may need your glasses or even a magnifying glass to read the markings. Since they are all designed with some differences, it is in your best interest to become familiar with the ones you usually take.

- Again, a simple strategy is for patients to have a copy of the phy-sician orders or the Medication Administration Record (MAR), which allows them to function as roadblocks for errors.

Learn the 10 *most lethal* medication errors:

1. Administering concentrated KCL

2. Errors in insulin dosing

3. Administration of intravenous calcium or magnesium

4. Inadvertent administration of 50 percent dextrose solution

5. Administering medications in spite of documented allergies

6. Miscalculated digoxin dosing in pediatric patients

7. Mixing up the chemotherapy drugs vincristine and vinblastine

8. Administering concentrated NaCL (sodium chloride)

9. Administering IV narcotic agents (morphine, dilaudid, fentanyl, etc.)

10. Errors in aminophylline dosing

According to the USP Medication Errors Reporting Program (MERP), almost *half* of all medication errors involve insulin. Realize that *only 10 drugs* account for over 60 percent of all adverse drug events.

- They are, in descending order of occurrence: the anticoagulants (blood thinners) warfarin and heparin; the opiate agonists morphine and meperidine; insulin; the benzodiazepine midazolam (Versed); digoxin, the anti-seizure drug phenytoin (Dilantin); the antibiotic cyclosporine; and promethazine (Phenergan).

- A quick checklist to confirm medication orders filled out by nurses before administering any medication would prevent many errors, so ask the staff to double-check all medications, and double-check for yourself on the flow sheet.

- If one day, you are given a pill that looks different from the pill you're used to taking, don't be afraid to ask why. A change in color, shape or size is a valid reason to alert the nurse. Simply ask, "This pill doesn't look like the one I've been taking. Is this right? Would you please phone the pharmacy to verify that this is the right medication and the correct dose?" It may all be above board; the hospital may simply use a different manufacturer than your pharmacy uses. But to be safe, be sure. Taking the time to ask a simple question could save your life.

- Drug compatibility must also be evaluated before drugs are administered. Many intravenous medications are incompatible with each other and cannot be mixed together in IV tubing. Incompatible medications that mix with each other in IV tubing can reduce the efficacy of one or more of the drugs or chemical reactions can occur, causing the drugs to form a precipitate and clog the IV line. If any of your drugs are incompatible, a saline flush needs to be given before infusing the second drug to ensure that the medications do not come into contact with each other.

- Ask if any of your medications are incompatible with each other, and be sure that a flush is used for IV solutions. You don't need any special knowledge about pharmaceuticals simply to ask, "Are you sure that all my IV medications are compatible with each other? I know that if certain drugs are given at the same time or even in close proximity there can be a problem." If there is any doubt, the pharmacist must be consulted. Other measures, like waiting a certain amount of time in between doses of certain classes of medications or avoiding dairy products, might be needed to prevent medication interactions. Have your nurse put a note on the IV pump or a label on the tubing to alert other staff members if any of your medications have compatibility issues.

- Be aware that elderly or debilitated relatives may not comprehend the importance of specific instructions about medications. The Institute for Safe Medication Practices (ISMP) reported on an 83-year-old woman who died from repeatedly chewing her Cardizem CD tablet instead of swallowing it whole. Cardizem CD is a sustained-release heart medication, and chewing the tablets can result in a fatal overdose.

- Realize that transdermal patches, which are commonly used to administer hormones, nicotine for smoking cessation programs, and narcotics for pain relief, are another potential source of medication errors. The most common problem is an overdose of medication when patients or their caregivers forget that a patch has been previously applied and then use another one. The FDA Patient Safety News reported cases in which patients died after several fentanyl patches for pain control were mistakenly applied to the skin simultaneously. If possible, avoid the use of clear patches, which are easier to forget about. If you are hospitalized, be sure the date, time, and location on the body that patches are applied to are recorded in your chart. If you are using transdermal patches at home, mark the date on a calendar you applied each patch. Lastly, if you are using a patch for pain relief you should know that heat can speed up the release of fentanyl from the patch, so avoid the use of heating pads, electric blankets, heat lamps, saunas, hot tubs and heated water beds while using a narcotic patch for pain control.

MONITORING RESPONSE

After the right drug has been administered, careful monitoring of the patient's response is essential; after all, every body is different. Even patients who have previously taken a medication without problems can one day, without warning, have an allergic reaction. If staff members do not recognize potentially serious medication reactions for what they are, then lifesaving interventions won't be initiated. In fact, nurses have less time than ever to monitor patients, so patients who are not responding well to a drug regimen can easily slip through the cracks.

Action Steps

- While you are receiving medications, careful monitoring will greatly reduce the likelihood of adverse events, so ask for it and expect it.

- Your response to a drug must be regularly evaluated and recorded in the medical record. Any adverse reactions should be noted in your chart, and you should document the fact for your records.

- If you have any adverse reactions or possible allergic reactions, you must be evaluated immediately. Patients not only have to be concerned about drugs; they can have allergic reactions to food, dyes used in diagnostic tests, adhesive tape, and the latex gloves worn by staff members.

- Report any reaction, no matter how minor, including itching, rash, hives, breathing difficulties, nausea or vomiting. An undiagnosed allergic reaction can lead to serious and even life-threatening complications, which require immediate attention. Patients can report reactions to vaccines by calling the Vaccine Adverse Events Reporting System (VAERS) at 1-800-822-7967 or fill out an online form at www.vaers.org.

- After you have started a medication regimen, it needs to be evaluated for efficacy. Is the drug working? How long will your doctor wait to see if it is? What other drugs can be used if this one proves ineffective? Proper monitoring will also include constant vigilance for drug interactions.

Confirming and Reporting Medication Errors

Medical patients are often unaware that a mistake has been made in their treatment or drug regimen because hospitals and doctors are not legally obligated to inform them of errors. Research conducted by ISMP in 1999 found that only 44 percent of medication errors that the respondents considered "serious" were disclosed to patients or to their family members. A research study published in 2000 in the journal *Archives of Disease in Childhood* reported that parents were told of medication errors involving their children only 48 percent of the time. The March 2002 issue of *Joint Commission Perspectives* revealed the shocking fact that when hospital staff members are involved in a medication error, most are never told about the mistake, depriving them of the vital information they need to avoid making the same mistake in the future. Patients who do realize that an error has occurred often have no idea how to respond or what action to take. Now you will know which aspects of medical treatment pose the greatest risk of errors and have the skills needed to protect yourself from harm. It is essential that you learn to identify, confirm, and report incidents that endanger their recovery. Here's what you should do:

Action Steps

- Know the three drug events that cause 50 percent of the reported medication errors: Overdose of anticoagulants (blood-thinning medications such as Coumadin or heparin); incorrect use of opiate agonists; inappropriate doses of insulin due to insufficient glucose monitoring.

- Ask your nurse, doctor, or a hospital administrator if you suspect that you have been involved in a medication mishap by asking point-blank, "Do you consider this event to be a medication error?" "Why or why not?"

- Patients who are given a narcotic reversal agent such as Narcan should be suspicious. This is often a sign that they have been overdosed with a narcotic medication and the situation is being remedied by the administration of another drug.

- The use of narcotic reversal agents such as Narcan should lead to the initiation of a review by the hospital. Insist on it.

If the staff confirms that a medication error has happened, be sure that the following steps are taken:

1. Your nurse should report the error immediately to the nursing supervisor and to the attending physician. If a nurse seems unwilling to do this, ask to speak directly to a supervisor.

2. The error should be noted in detail in your medical record.

3. Ask the nurse to fill out an Occurrence Report or an Adverse Drug Event Reporting Form. Hospitals may have different names for these forms, but when you use this terminology they'll know what you are referring to.

4. If the error involves the pharmacy, the nurse should notify the pharmacist. If the wrong drug or the wrong dose was sent from the pharmacy, they need to know immediately in order to assess the systems error that allowed the wrong medication to reach the floor and to prevent other patients from receiving medications in error.

5. Tell the nursing supervisor or the attending physician that you want the medication error to be reported to the USP-ISMP Medication Errors Reporting Program (MERP). USP is U.S. Pharmacopeia, and ISMP is the Institute for Safe Medication Practices. Staff members can make confidential reports to the MERP program by calling 1-800-23-ERROR or through the Internet at www.usp.org. While doing research interviews for this book, a spokeswoman for the MERP program informed me that patients can also use this reporting service. Report all

medication errors, even near misses, by calling the above 800 number. This information is entered into a database to track errors, and the FDA and the drug manufacturer can be alerted that an error, or even a close call, has occurred. Patients can check the Internet sites www.ismp.org and www.usp.org for information on medication errors.

Additional Areas of Risk

PATIENT INJURIES

Anyone entering the hospital naturally feels some degree of apprehension about his treatment and recovery. In addition to the obvious concerns about the risks of anesthesia, surgery, or infection, all patients must be cognizant of the fact that *every* person who enters the hospital is at risk for being injured in an accident. Patient injuries from accidents are an ongoing problem in our hospitals and often result in a permanent loss of some function. Risk managers consistently rank patient falls as one of the top 10 liabilities faced by hospitals.

In 1996, the Superior Court of New Jersey upheld a 1.6 million-dollar malpractice award to a man who fell out of his hospital bed as he desperately tried to reach the call button. The man had been injured in a motor vehicle accident and had a trache tube inserted in his throat to help him breathe. The tube became obstructed by mucus, and the patient was unable to call for help because the tracheostomy procedure left him temporarily unable to speak. One can only imagine his panic and terror as he frantically reached for the call button—grasping for his only chance at survival. The patient, found on the floor, sustained head trauma and a broken hip. The court ruled that it was negligent to leave this patient alone for 30 minutes and that leaving the patient without easy access to his call button did not meet basic standard of care criteria.

FALLS

Falls consistently make the top 10 lists for patient injuries that often result in lawsuits. While most people naturally assume that the elderly are at the greatest risk of falling, the median age of people injured in falls is actually only 58. Most falls happen in the patient's room or bathroom while she is all alone. One of the major contributing factors in these accidents is that the staff has not properly assessed each individual patient's risk of falling and then taken the right precautions. And whenever there are fewer nurses working a particular shift, it means that there is less observation and supervision. Another problem is the use of agency nurses who are unfamiliar with the patients and possibly unacquainted with hospital protocols for preventing accidents. Finally, there is the lack of communication among staff about individual patient needs.

Action Steps

- Be informed of the basic safety precautions for preventing injuries from falls. Don't assume that keeping the bed rails up will prevent one. In fact, research suggests that using bed rails may actually increase agitation levels in some patients and can result in a greater number of injuries when the patient, in panic, tries to climb over the rails.

- Know what conditions put you at a greater risk for falls. High-risk groups include the elderly, small children, people with limited mobility, people with mental impairment and patients using medications such as narcotics or sleep aids.

- Realize that a bed or wheelchair that moves can cause you to lose your balance and fall, so be sure that the wheels are always locked.

- Wet floors present another obvious risk for patients, so be aware of spills.

- If you are unsteady on your feet, you should have a walker available to assist you and a commode or urinal next to your bed, so you don't have to walk to the bathroom. The bedside table, the controls for the bed and television, the telephone, the call button, and your glasses should be within easy reach at all times.

- Inspect the rubber tips on canes, crutches, and walkers to be sure that they are intact and not excessively worn.

- You are at an increased risk for tumbling onto the floor if you are on a gurney or an x-ray table, so be extra careful in those locations.

- Any medication that makes you dizzy, sleepy, or nauseated should put you on alert. Ask about the side effects of any pre-scription drug you are ingesting, or take a proactive approach and look them up for yourself in the drug reference book you have brought with you to the hospital. If you are taking diuret-ics, you don't want to be in such a hurry to reach the bathroom that you break your leg on the way.

- Realize that you are likely to feel stressed in the hospital, which may hinder your sleep; drowsiness makes people less attentive to obstacles. Although it is tempting to ask for sleep aids, the hospital is probably not a good place to try a sleep medication for the first time. The sleep aid may interact with other medica-tions you are taking and may make you a little ungainly. Get lots of rest prior to hospitalization, and plan on catching up on your sleep at home.

- Don't think that just because you aren't old or feeble, you can't take a tumble doing the simplest thing in the hospital. Just know that it's a lot easier than you think. Talk to the staff about your side effects and reactions to medications, and have a friend or relative stay with you as much as possible—preferably 24 hours a day.

HOSPITAL BED SAFETY

Between 1985 and 2006, the FDA received 691 reports of patients becoming entrapped in bed rails, with a significant number causing the patient's death. These figures include only the accidents reported to the FDA—it is generally accepted that the numbers are actually much higher. A number of deaths involved air mattresses. Air mattresses can be built in features of a bed, or they can be placed on top of regular hospital mattress. Elderly patients with fragile skin are often placed on air mattresses to relieve pressure on parts of their bodies prone to bedsores, so they are particularly prone to this problem. Other known entrapments are gaps between the mattress and the bed rails or bed frames that are too large; these conditions allow patient's head to become trapped. Patient's heads have also been caught in between the bed rails, and vest-type restraints have led to them becoming entangled in the rails.

Action Steps

* Be aware that elderly patients, immobile patients, heavily medicated patients, patients with mental impairment, and patients who are restrained are at increased risk for becoming ensnared in their beds. Any medication that makes you dizzy or sleepy should put you on alert.

* Evaluate your own hospital bed closely when you check in. The mattress should fit the bed frame snugly and not slide easily. The mattress should be the right size for the frame, with less than a 4¾ inch gap between a compressed mattress and the frame. The spaces between the rails should also be less than 4¾ inches. If your mattress or rail does not meet the above criteria, insist on a different bed.

* Ask for anti-skid mats or even strips of Velcro under the air mattresses if they are to be placed on top of regular mattresses; this is to keep the air mattress from sliding or moving which can create a gap on one side that can lead to asphyxiation if the patient rolls over into the gap.

* Determine whether the bed rails should be kept up for you or your loved one. If they are left up, remember that they're considered a "restraint system," and therefore care must be taken

with their use. Bed rails can be fitted with netting-type covers to prevent entrapments. Nurses must be able to see through any bed rail cover to be able to observe the patient, so don't prop pillows or blankets next to the rails if the patient will be left alone.

- If you or a loved one have a condition that necessitates assistance for every minor activity or need constant supervision due to mental impairment from a diagnosis such as dementia, realize that most hospitals are not in a position to provide it. Patients in intensive care units will have their own nurse to see to their every need, but patients on regular floors will not receive this amount of attention. A family member or advocate must make the commitment to stay with you and aid in your supervision.

- Anticipate needs such as having to visit the bathroom frequently, thirst, boredom, etc. Try to find solutions to these issues in advance.

- Visit the VHA National Center for Patient Safety website at www.visn8.med.va.gov/patientsafetycenter and click on Hospital Bed Safety to print up "A Guide to Bed Safety for Patients and Families" or phone (813) 558-3911 for guidance.

INTRAVENOUS LINES

Intravenous lines can be the cause of injuries that range from mild to severe. Examples of minor injuries are slight bruising or transient swelling, which is merely an uncomfortable nuisance. Fluid from IV lines may infiltrate blood vessels, causing pain, moderate swelling, and the need to remove the line and stick the patient again at a new site. More seriously, IV lines can be a source of deadly bloodstream infections and blood clots. Careful insertion technique and vigilant monitoring of IV lines by both healthcare workers and patients can make IV therapy successful, which essentially means that it is uneventful.

Action Steps

- You or your advocate must alert your caregiver if you notice any pain, swelling, moistness, redness, itching, or bruising at your IV site.

- Ring for the nurse when your IV pump alarms, so the line does not remain static for any length of time.

- As annoying as the sound of the alarm might be, resist the temptation to push the button to silence the alarm on your pump. The alarm is signaling for a reason and it is easy to forget that you pushed the button once it is quiet. Do not tamper in any way with your infusion pump.

- Report blood backing up into the tubing, since this can indicate that a clamp needs to be opened or it can be a signal of an inadequate infusion rate.

- IV lines that are still in place but not being used might need to be flushed with an appropriate blood thinner such as heparin; ask your nurse or doctor. IV catheters that remain static too long may form blood clots that can render the line useless and endanger your health.

- IVs should be removed when they are no longer needed. Ask regularly if it's time to take out your line.

EQUIPMENT AND DEVICE PROBLEMS

Medical equipment and devices are no less prone to mechanical failure than any other of our high-tech advances. The devices we count on to save our lives routinely malfunction, break down, are programmed incorrectly and contain poorly designed safety features. I read regularly about prosthetic joints being recalled, pacemakers malfunctioning, IV pumps delivering deadly amounts of medications, and alarms failing to alert staff to life-threatening fluctuations in vital signs. With careful observation, you can thwart a significant number of mishaps.

EQUIPMENT IMPROPERLY MAINTAINED, PROGRAMMED, OR UTILIZED

In 2001, the FDA reported that 28 patients at the Panama National Institute of Oncology were overexposed to radiation during their cancer treatments. The overexposures ranged from 20 percent to a startling 100 percent over the ordered dose, all from machines that were improperly programmed. Five deaths were attributed to the radiation overexposure, and the remaining patients are at risk of developing serious radiation-related complications.

In December of 2000, four women died of asphyxiation when a nursing home employee erroneously hooked up a nitrogen tank to the oxygen system. The fitting on the nitrogen tank was not compatible with the oxygen delivery system, which should have clued him in immediately that something wasn't right. Instead of questioning why the fitting was incompatible, however, and calling for help, the employee, on his own, removed a fitting from another oxygen tank and jury-rigged it to the nitrogen tank. He later argued that the tanks looked identical, that the supply company was not supposed to deliver nitrogen to the nursing home, and that an oxygen label had been only partially covered by a nitrogen label. Medical equipment poses risks to patients in a number of ways: labeling, maintenance, programming, or usage.

Action Steps

- As obvious as it may seem, you need to be sure that the machines used in your care are plugged in and working. Most of the time, looking at the numbers on the display to be sure that they are changing is a good indicator that the device is at least running. Check every plug, every piece of tubing, and every monitor. I've observed staff move patients into a room with the prongs of their oxygen mask in their nose and forget to connect the tubing to the wall outlet, putting the patient into oxygen deficit.

- Ask the nurse to verify that all alarm features are functioning and are set at an audible level. The staff has to be able to hear them from outside your room.

- You and your loved ones should know the dose of radiation that you are receiving, ask who will be programming the machine, and be sure that someone verifies the correct numbers on the control panel.

- If you are a radiation or chemotherapy patient, insist that the dosages of your treatments be verified by a second set of calculations, since errors at this stage can cause serious damage.

- Regular servicing will reduce the number of machines that fail to operate properly. All machines used in hospitals should have a sticker in a clearly visible area that gives the date that the machine was last serviced and the date that service will be needed again. Look for it, and make sure it is up to date.

- Ask that device malfunctions be documented by the staff, that the defective machine be removed from service, and that it be properly labeled so it will not be used on another patient.

- Be aware that MRI machines utilize an electromagnet powerful enough to cause metal objects to fly through the room. Be sure there are no metal objects on or around you before you enter the room. In 2001, a six-year old boy was killed when an oxygen tank struck him in the head as it was pulled towards the magnet in the MRI machine. In another instance, a police officer who stepped inside a MRI scanning room to guard a prisoner had his gun ripped out of his holster by the force of the magnet. Don't underestimate the danger of flying metal objects; even objects as small as a piece of jewelry or a metal hair clip have caused serious injuries as they were hurled around a room.

Mistakes that occur due to inexperience, fatigue or carelessness violate our trust since patients are entitled to be protected by the primary rule of medicine: First, do no harm. There is no justification for the public being treated by healthcare workers who are impaired by substance abuse, untreated mental illness, a simple lack of sleep, or poor training.

Mental fatigue and outright illness both play roles in medical errors. Recently in Boston, a surgeon left his patient on the operating room table half way through back surgery because he wanted to get to the bank on time to make a deposit. It was later determined that he was suffering from mental illness, which, hopefully, we can identify earlier if people start paying closer attention to their colleagues. Hospital administrators and physicians find it discomforting to approach staff members or peers who are exhibiting odd behavior because emotional stress is a touchy subject with people. But by not doing it, they actually fail their colleagues and leave the lives of patients hanging in the balance. Unrealistic work schedules have been an obvious culprit for years now in creating emotional stress. Hospital administrators know this, but the moment the financial reality of hiring more staff is on the table, real reform comes to a standstill.

Why is it that no other industry has adopted an operating strategy in which their employees work 80 to 120 hours a week for a nominal salary? Because recruiting and retaining good employees would be nearly impossible, and the prognosis for long-term success would be dim. Why don't other industries try out inexperienced personnel on the unsuspecting public? You don't see novice airline pilots, for instance, being told to prove themselves worthy of their license by flying a plane full of passengers across the Atlantic Ocean. Why not? Because it is reckless and dangerous. But this is exactly what we do in medicine with our "watch one, do one, teach one" philosophy. Who in his right mind would assign a first-year medical resident with virtually no experience to manage a busy emergency room in the middle of the night? The employees themselves are frustrated, and the quality of their performance may suffer. Certainly, their salary and treatment do not motivate them to rise above the circumstances and do a better job; only unstinting devotion to a higher purpose accomplishes that. To date, we have seen each of these problems rear its ugly head in healthcare, and as long as the problems continue unchecked, they pave the way for a medical system on a collision course for financial red ink, healthcare rationing, and a rising death toll.

INCOMPETENT PHYSICIANS AND THOSE WITH MEDICAL BOARD CENSURES

Doctors can be incompetent, negligent, addicted to drugs, or suffering from mental illnesses that render them dangerous to their patients. A Manhattan obstetrician delivered a healthy baby girl and then carved his initials into the mother's stomach just for the heck of it. The doctor's attorney blamed a frontal lobe disorder for the doctor's unstable behavior. Chemical dependency is one of the most frequent causes of disability among physicians, and substance abuse is the most common form of impairment disciplined by state medical boards. Statistics continue to show that physicians are prone to the same vulnerabilities to drugs and alcohol as the general public and at roughly the same rates, but their indulgences can cause great harm. Americans have a lifetime risk of substance abuse of 14.6 percent, meaning that almost 15 percent of us will, at some point, abuse illicit drugs or alcohol. It is estimated that 7 percent of practicing physicians in this country are substance abusers, which equates to 1 in every 14 doctors. The numbers remain steady across geographical location, specialty, age and type of practice. With approximately 800,000 physicians in the United States, 56,000 will struggle with addictive tendencies at some point in their career.

Action Steps

- Check your doctor's credentials on the Internet by accessing the website of your state medical board.

- During your visit to your physician, ask specific questions to discern all pertinent information about his or her level of expertise. How long has he been in practice? How many procedures like yours has she performed, and what is her success rate?

- If the doctor is a specialist, is she board certified in her specialty?

- Does your doctor track her statistics to determine if her patients are developing hospital-acquired infections? Does she follow up on her infection statistics and look for innovative ways to reduce her infection rates?

- Will the doctor be using an unfamiliar piece of equipment or a new technique? If so, how many hours of hands-on training has she received?

INEXPERIENCE

It is common for relatively inexperienced physicians to be left in charge of emergency rooms or patient units, especially in the middle of the night. The first doctor to respond to your health needs may well be the one with the least amount of experience. Inexperienced staff members may also be allowed to perform invasive procedures without the direct supervision of an attending physician—shocking but true. These individuals are not bad doctors; they're just green. They are being pressured to do something before they're ready, and it can be disastrous for their patients.

Action Steps

- Know the facts about who will be caring for you and their level of expertise. See Chapter Two - The Health Care Team.

- A thorough pre-operative visit is important to allow you to meet your surgeon and to ask questions about his or her experience with your procedure.

- If you are a patient in a teaching hospital, you do not have to be cared for by someone who is unqualified, *even if you have signed consent forms allowing residents to participate in your care.*

- Residents may resist doing this, but know that if you feel uneasy about the decisions made on your behalf, a more experienced physician can always be consulted – even in the middle of the night.

SLEEP DEPRIVATION AND EXCESSIVE FATIGUE

European researchers have reported that babies born between the hours of 9 p.m. and 6:59 a.m. are almost twice as likely to die in the first few weeks of life as compared to infants born during the day. Even more alarming was the fact that the researchers identified medical personnel fatigue during night shifts as a significant contributing factor. Individuals who are sleep-deprived often exhibit clumsiness, blurred vision, decreased reflexes and response time, flawed reasoning and judgment ability, confusion, and irritability – not exactly desirable qualities for someone charged with an important job. The British journal, *Nature*, reported in 1997 that staying awake for 24 hours leaves a person in a state comparable to someone with a blood alcohol level of .10 – legally drunk in most states.

Excessive amounts of fatigue and sleep deprivation are still benchmarks of medical training, even though everyone knows the practice puts patient's lives at risk. It has been the norm for medical residents to work in excess of 80 to 100 hours per week. The Patient and Physician Protection Act of 2001 was introduced to limit residents to an 80- hour workweek and to ensure that shifts do not exceed 24 hours. Starting July 2003, the Accreditation Council for Graduate Medical Education will adopt standards that limit residents to work no more than 80 hours a week, but averaged over *a four-week* period, so a certain week could involve working more than 80 hours. Under the Patient and Physician Safety and Protection Act of 2005, which has not yet been passed into law, emergency rooms, which have a higher rate of error, would be required to limit residents to 12-hour shifts, and residents could only be on call one night out of every three and are required to have one day out of seven off. It's hard to believe that this modified work schedule, which is still grueling, is considered to be a progressive, even radical, change in medical education.

Action Steps

- You do not have to be treated by staff members who are impaired by fatigue. Expect your healthcare providers to be alert and competent at all times, no matter what hour of the day it is.

- Don't jeopardize your life by ignoring signs of sleep deprivation. You wouldn't think twice about speaking up if one of your doctors reeked of alcohol, so why tolerate their fatigue when it can represent the same risk to your health? Notify the nursing supervisor, the Patient Relations department, and the hospital administrator as soon as you suspect that any staff members are excessively fatigued, and ask that the responsibility of your care be transferred to a well-rested provider.

- If the problem persists, write your own entry to be added to your medical record to document your alarm about the fatigue level you are witnessing (See Chapter 7). The chart entry should include your name, the date and time, a brief explanation of your concern, and the names of the individuals you alerted to the situation.

Chapter Five

Second Opinions

Not everyone truly appreciates the value of second opinions, but after dealing with my daughter's many ordeals in the health-care system, my husband and I became not just believers, but apostles. As you will see in this chapter, seeking a second opinion will almost certainly offer peace of mind and reduce fears about a course of action, but it could also save your life.

After years of involvement, we grew so adept at interacting with all facets of the system that we became a resource for family, friends and coworkers. One weekend my husband, who is a police officer, received an emergency page from another officer named Steve, who had just heard that he'd been diagnosed with stomach cancer. He was a young, physically fit and dedicated police officer who was expecting his second child. The devastating news about his health could hardly have come at a worse time.

Everything was to move very quickly; he was scheduled to have his stomach removed the following week, barely allowing enough time to process the new information. The first evidence that he had a problem was an incident in which he had doubled over with stomach pain so severe that he was rushed to the emergency room, where he was given acid-reducing medications and then scheduled for an endoscopy: the doctor inserts a scope into the stomach to evaluate its appearance and take small tissue biopsies. After the procedure, Steve's doctor expressed concern about the appearance of the tissue samples, but interjected that only a pathologist could offer a definite answer about whether Steve had a malignancy. The patient was released from the hospital the next day and simply told to wait. He continued to take the acid-reducing medication and was encouraged to find that his symptoms improved.

He was so optimistic that he began to think the biopsy would confirm nothing more than an ulcer, which wasn't an uncommon affliction for a type-A, hard-charging police officer. Unfortunately, a few days later, the doctor phoned and gave him the worst possible diagnosis: a highly invasive stomach cancer that would require immediate surgery, and possibly other therapies like chemotherapy and radiation. Steve was referred to a surgeon for a pre-surgical consultation, where he was told that he would have to remove his entire stomach if he wanted the best chance of survival. As he sat there watching a complete stranger diagram his stomach and deliver news that would change his life forever—as calmly as if she were presenting a weather report—he suddenly realized that he needed to slow the process down. *This is all going too fast,* he thought.

Before he would consent to surgery that would remove an organ as important as his stomach, he decided that a second opinion was in order. That is when he came to us. My husband told him to get a copy of his pathology report and referred him to an oncologist we knew and trusted. This oncologist requested the pathology slides—not just the report, which is what the surgeon saw when she made her decision—and showed them to a pathologist he worked with at a medical center in San Francisco. After the new pathologist read the report and reviewed the slides, he came to a startling conclusion: there wasn't nearly enough information to make a diagnosis as drastic as stomach cancer because there was so much inflammation in Steve's stomach lining, it could have caused a false report. Thus, the biopsy samples could not be counted on to say for certain that cancer cells were present. Steve was put on a regimen of acid-reducing medications for a month to reduce the inflammation, at which time a reliable endoscopy would be performed. Needless to say, it was an arduous month.

The second biopsy revealed that Steve had a severe ulcer, not cancer. When the original pathologist was informed of his error, the man admitted that he had felt "pressured" by the doctor to diagnose cancer. Apparently, when the surgeon had delivered the tissue specimens to the lab, he announced, "This is definitely cancer." He insisted on a quick diagnosis because "this guy needs surgery right away if he's to have any chance at all." The pathologist expressed his misgivings about the quality of the tissue sample but was assured by the doctor that what he had seen through the scope was indeed cancer. The pathologist, who somewhat excused himself by saying that the deck had been stacked against his own opinion, did apologize for the near miss.

Here we have a case of a doctor influencing a hesitant pathologist. When he was questioned about the quality of the tissue specimen, the doctor resorted to the old standby, "I've seen enough cases of cancer to know one when I see it." Both of these people were well intentioned, but if left unchecked, they would have set into motion a series of events that would have had disastrous consequences for their patient. Steve could have been condemned to spend the rest of his life without a stomach and forced to ingest his nutrition through a tube.

I am sorry to say that stories like this are not uncommon. In a 1999 study of 6,000 patients published in *Cancer*, it was reported that of all the people who came to a certain large medical center following a biopsy, one to two people out of every one hundred had received a "totally wrong" diagnosis. The culprits were both hospitals and laboratories, with 86 patients out of 6,000 being misdiagnosed. Dr. Jonathon L. Epstein, one of the authors of the study, actually called some of the errors "harrowing." A percentage of 1.4 may seem small, but remember, if you are in that group, the odds will suddenly appear astronomical.

You might, of course, be lucky like Steve mentioned above, but you cannot count on it. In 2003, the *New England Journal of Medicine* published the results of a two-year Rand Corporation study illustrating that patients receive the correct diagnosis and treatment, for a variety of common medical conditions, only 55 percent of the time! The comprehensive study included 13,000 patient interviews and a review of 6,712 medical records, and it is worth going into in some detail because it reveals so much about the value of second opinions.

The startling statistics presented in the Rand study clearly illustrate the benefits of having another doctor review your diagnosis and treatment plan. You want to be sure that you are receiving exactly the right care for a particular ailment. Sometimes the problem with consulting only one doctor is that an easy, almost cost-free therapy could have been employed and patients simply weren't informed. In the above study, 40 percent of the participants with heart problems could have benefited from aspirin therapy, but their doctors never told them they should use it. Imagine enduring a second heart attack or a stroke just because you didn't know enough to take an over-the-counter medication that costs a nickel.

Of all the patients with high blood pressure, a full 35 percent weren't properly diagnosed or given the correct dose of medication to control their disease and avoid a potential stroke. And a shocking 75 percent of diabetics weren't receiving the recommended blood sugar testing to assess the effectiveness of their medication. This is serious because even a small elevation in blood sugar, if allowed to become a chronic state for a diabetic patient, can lead to devastating complications. A check by a physician or a nurse who specializes in the care and education of diabetic patients may lead to modifications in a testing schedule or in the dose of insulin, which can make all the difference.

Another group that was at risk was elderly patients. Only 64 percent had been offered a pneumonia vaccine, which meant they were exposed to greater odds of dying from complications of an illness that strikes the elderly population particularly hard. An older patient, especially one with several medical conditions or who is taking multiple medications, may want to consult a physician who specializes in geriatric care. Even people just over 50 need to be careful. Only 38 percent of participants over that age had been screened for colon cancer, even though we now know that early detection increases the odds of survival by a substantial margin.

Heart patients must be especially vigilant in our healthcare system. The Agency for Healthcare Research and Quality (AHRQ) reports that only 21 percent of eligible elderly patients receive beta blockers following a heart attack, despite proof that these drugs have the ability to reduce deaths by 43 percent. Beta blocker usage increased 63 percent after hospitals and physicians were alerted to the problem—proof of how easily some of these dangers can be remedied! If you, or someone you love, suffer from a serious condition such as heart disease, make sure you look into the most up-to-date medical research. Personally, I would never trust my care to a single cardiologist without the input from a second heart specialist to confirm that my treatment was absolutely top notch. If there is a pill that I can take to reduce my chances of dying by 43 percent, then I want to hear about it. I certainly don't want to be left out in the cold just because I was in the group of eligible heart patients who simply wasn't told about beta blockers.

The above statistics prove that you cannot just sit back and wait for your busy physician automatically to order every screening test or necessary medication at the exactly the right time. There are books, the Internet, and health fairs to take advantage of in your quest to play an active part in your own care. Check www.hospitalcompare.hhs.gov for information about your hospital's statistics regarding compliance with dozens of recommended care standards for heart attacks, heart failure, pneumonia and surgery. If your hospital is deficient in any area, you need to be all the more vigilant. Print out the graph and bring it with you to the hospital to be sure nothing is missed. And don't forget to pay attention to the experiences of your friends. It is probably not just a coincidence that all your friends approximately your own age are having colonoscopies or mammograms. If your doctor won't follow through, or shrugs off your need for any test or medication that is suggested by current standards, that is a sure sign that it is time to consult someone else.

I've met people who think there is a cut-off date for seeking the opinion of another doctor. Every patient has the right to seek one *at any time* during their treatment—beginning, middle or end. Another misconception is that a second opinion is sought only in life and death situations or for "bad news" diagnoses. Sometimes you simply need one for your own peace of mind or to validate what you are sensing about your own condition. A case in point is that of Laura Hillenbrand, the best-selling author of the book *Seabiscuit*. Fourteen years ago, Ms. Hillenbrand went to her doctor with baffling symptoms. She was a young, healthy 19-year-old girl who, out of nowhere, had begun to complain of fever, vertigo, fatigue, swollen lymph nodes, weight loss, hair loss, night sweats, and sores in her mouth and throat. In the years that followed, these symptoms were diagnosed as bulimia, strep throat, Epstein-Barr, food poisoning and depression. One physician actually suggested that the straight-A student was only trying to get out of going to class. Not one of these felt true to her. Finally, a doctor who was in the infectious disease department at Johns Hopkins Hospital gave her a diagnosis: Chronic Fatigue Syndrome. He couldn't offer her a cure or even much in the way of therapeutic treatment. Nevertheless, his words came as a relief because "to finally get a diagnosis, to finally have someone be compassionate and take me seriously, was an enormous event."

If there are so many obvious benefits to seeking second opinions, why don't more people do it? One of the biggest obstacles is the patient's fear of offending his present doctor. However, a truly competent physician will welcome another point of view by a colleague, and he will respect his patient's right to make her own decision. Confident physicians want their patients to be informed.

Second opinions are warranted for a number of reasons. The following is a list of the most important, and therefore the ones I will cover in this chapter:

1. When an uncertain or unconfirmed diagnosis could lead to the wrong treatment plan

2. When there is a diagnosis of a serious, rare, or life-threatening illness

3. When a treatment plan is unacceptable to you

4. When you want to explore other treatment options

5. When a prescribed treatment is not working for you

6. When you aren't feeling that you are part of the team

7. When your doctor has an operating style or decision-making style that is out of sync with your own

8. When you have a problem with the doctor's level of experience, competence or ethics

9. When there is a difference in philosophy about when to continue treatment or end treatment

10. When your intuition is telling you that something just isn't right

An Uncertain or Unconfirmed Diagnosis that Could Lead to the Wrong Treatment Plan

An accurate diagnosis is vital to the formation of an appropriate plan. Nobody wants treatment they don't need, or to be deprived of treatment they do need. If your physician is unsure of her diagnosis, if there are questions about the "staging" of a malignancy or disease, or if your own intuition is causing you to doubt the diagnosis, check with another doctor. You can save yourself precious time as well as physical and emotional resources by avoiding a treatment that has no chance at all of being successful. If you have any disagreement with your doctor or doubts about your diagnosis, you need to consult another physician.

The following is a list of circumstances related to the diagnostic process that would justify seeking a second opinion:

1. Your physician is unsure about your diagnosis

2. Your biopsy results are inconclusive

3. Several tests you have already completed need to be repeated in order to firm up a diagnosis

4. There are questions about the "staging" of a malignancy or disease

5. Your intuition leaves you with nagging doubts about your diagnosis.

As we can see from Steve's story, even pathology results don't necessarily provide hard and fast answers. You could easily be lulled into believing that when a doctor examines your cells through a microscope, he cannot possibly misinterpret what he sees, but pathology is considered as much an art as a science. Often, there are subtle nuances in cells that lead one pathologist to one conclusion and another to a completely different determination.

If you are ever presented with frightening pathology results, make sure the diagnosis is absolutely accurate. Every step you take from that moment forward depends on it. Toward that end, these are some of the steps you can take to help assure its accuracy:

1. It is extremely important to ask if a second pathologist has confirmed your results. Hopefully, the hospital that performed your biopsy has a policy requiring all biopsy results to be reviewed and confirmed by a second pathologist, but you must ask. If this is not its usual procedure, ask that it be done for you.

2. If you are told that you must have a second biopsy performed, it could be an indication that a better sample was needed in the first place. Confirm that the surgeon has conferred with the pathologist in advance to be sure that the new specimen is appropriate for the pathologist's needs. The lab might need a larger piece of tissue or have a special requirement for preserving the sample as it is being obtained.

3. It is not unusual at the time of a cancer diagnosis for tumors to be present in two or more organs, which may make it extremely difficult to tell which one is the "primary," or original, tumor. It is vital to determine the site of the original tumor, since all treatment protocols will be based on the best form of therapy for that type of cancer. If you are told that you have malignancies in more than one location, a second look by a different pathologist is a must.

4. Consult an independent pathology group to review your slides and offer its diagnosis. Before agreeing to start a treatment protocol that includes the potentially life-threatening and irreversible complications that so often accompany surgery, chemotherapy, radiation, or amputation, I would strongly urge you to consider a second opinion on your pathology specimen. Note the resources listed at the end of this chapter for second opinions on pathology specimens that patients can obtain on their own.

Even after a definitive diagnosis has been made, you cannot become complacent because there could still be other nuances or characteristics that need to be interpreted by a pathologist. Using breast cancer as an example, even after the type and stage of the breast cancer has been determined, information about tumor markers, genetic mutations in the breast cancer gene, and whether or not the tumor cells are estrogen-dependent is needed from the pathologist. A scan of a cancer patient may show signs of lymph node involvement but the number of affected nodes and the depth of penetration of the cancerous cells cannot be definitively determined until they are biopsied. The aggressiveness of the treatment of many cancers is partially dependent on the amount of lymph node involvement, so you need to be sure. Your diagnostic information may place you in a gray area as to whether you should have adjunctive therapies, such as chemotherapy or radiation, in addition to surgery. No one wants more treatment than he or she needs, but you certainly don't want less treatment, since the first attempt at treating diseases like cancer often gives the greatest odds of success.

There is a Diagnosis of a Serious, Rare, or Life-threatening Illness

The diagnosis and treatment of a chronic, rare, or life-threatening illness are more complex than other diseases, and patients should always confer with a doctor who is a recognized specialist in that particular illness to increase the chance of receiving up-to-date treatment. Yet don't feel that you have to rely on only one doctor to handle all aspects of your treatment plan. Often, serious diseases require a team of specialists, and a multi-disciplinary approach (meaning many specialists) is called for. There is one situation in which seeking a second opinion is a must: if you have been given no hope of survival or offered no treatment plan except for pain relief.

In 1978, Richard Bloch, the founder of H&R Block, was diagnosed with terminal lung cancer and told that he had three months to live. Under those circumstances, he did not hesitate to obtain a second opinion because, "You have one chance to beat cancer. If you don't take advantage of it, there is no second chance." On the advice of another physician at MD Anderson Cancer Center, Bloch underwent a grueling two-year treatment regimen that included extensive lung surgery, chemotherapy and radiation. After the treatment proved successful, Bloch and his wife started the R.A. Bloch Cancer Foundation because he saw so clearly that patients needed help and guidance. *Twenty-five years* after his seemingly hopeless **diagnosis, Bloch** was still devoting his life to helping others. Bloch died in 2004 at age 78 of heart failure. To reach his foundation's toll-free **hotline, either** for information or to request a free copy of *Fighting Cancer*, one of three books published by Richard and Annette Bloch, call 1-800-433-0464. You can also check their Web site at www.blochcancer.org.

Whenever you are dealing with life-threatening and rare or serious conditions, a safe and moderate approach is not always the best course. Minimal risk sometimes spells out minimal chance of a cure. Some doctors are more aggressive than others, and you cannot assume that whichever physician you've ended up with will fight the way you want him to or arrive at a treatment plan that is perfectly suited to you. When the diagnosis is very serious, the doctor has to be open to a wider range of choices than if the illness is not life-threatening. Some doctors work only within a very narrow comfort zone, and you won't know if he is limiting your options in that way unless you do your homework. Ask your doctor who is in the "opposite camp" from him. Are there other doctors or medical centers that would treat your disease in a very different way? What institutions are conducting cutting-edge research or have specialized programs for patients with your condition? It is very easy to do an Internet search to look for doctors who are recognized experts for your condition. I have had great success phoning and/or emailing physicians all over the country to avail myself of their expertise. These experts are used to being contacted and are usually very responsive to patient inquiries. You can conduct your own Internet search or pay for a professional literature search for your diagnosis (see Chapter Four). And you may want to consider traveling out of state for a cure. The doctors at the University of California may have a completely different approach than those at Duke University across the country.

It is entirely possible that the next physician you consult will only validate what your original doctor said, but if you are about to undergo challenging or painful treatment, don't you want to be sure that no other course is open to you? A second look may just bring you peace of mind that comes from knowing you've exhausted all reasonable options, but that is no small thing. And, of course, it could also save your life.

A Treatment Plan That is Unacceptable to the Patient

Patients can object to a treatment plan because it is too aggressive or because it isn't aggressive enough. An 80-year old man with a slow-growing prostate malignancy may not want to put himself through strenuous chemotherapy and may opt for a less rigorous course of treatment, or no treatment at all. Some individuals feel that they want the time they have left to be unburdened by ongoing medical treatments or a series of hospitalizations. Some people need a treatment that, if they survive, will allow them to return to their previous lifestyle. Lance Armstrong, for instance, asked his oncologist to modify his treatment to give him the greatest chance of being able to return to competitive cycling. Lance's customized "back on the bike" treatment plan included brain surgery to remove two small lesions instead of using radiation on his brain, which could have resulted in memory and balance problems. And Armstrong had one of the standard chemotherapy agents for testicular cancer, bleomycin, eliminated after the first round because it is known to cause pulmonary toxicity, which almost certainly would have reduced the lung capacity necessary to compete in the Tour de France. This man had very compelling reasons to select a plan that minimized certain side effects.

Whenever a treatment plan involves irrevocable decisions, like amputation, you want to give it the most careful consideration and time before settling on a choice. If the treatment is wrong, you're the one who has to live with the consequences for the rest of your life. Another situation that warrants a careful look is when you have to try a medication that has potentially serious side effects. At least with medication, you have time to monitor your response and stop the plan if the effects are too noxious. With an amputation, a hysterectomy or the termination of a pregnancy, when it's done, it's done.

You can't change your mind later. The sheer number of stories in the media of, for instance, women who were advised to terminate their pregnancies to save their lives, only to defy conventional wisdom with successful results, is enough to make anyone get a second opinion. These women bravely defied their doctors' recommendations, delivered healthy babies, and survived their medical conditions. There are just as many stories about patients who refused to have diseased or damaged limbs amputated and went on to recover with their limbs intact. Of course, a serious case of gangrene may be insurmountable, but some patients may be willing to assume a higher level of risk and live with significant compromises in their mobility in order to avoid amputation. It can be risky to go against a doctor's opinion, even when another doctor backs you up, but as an individual you have to evaluate what is important to you. That which is acceptable to the doctor might be completely unacceptable to the patient.

Patients who are told that there is nothing else to be done about their condition always have to look elsewhere, even if only to confirm that nothing has been overlooked. A wait-and-see approach may be unacceptable to a patient who feels strongly that her condition is more serious than it appears to medical professionals. In some cases, patients may believe that a treatment plan is being steered by a certain interpretation of symptoms and not a definitive diagnostic test. In this case, they might wish to insist on a test or to see a specialist to find out if he would recommend the test. When symptoms are worsening, this step is even more important.

Even for non-serious conditions, patients often want more information. Those who haven't yet had diagnostic scans (such as a MRI) may not want to embark on a strenuous course of physical therapy or an exercise program that may actually exacerbate their condition. I know of this firsthand when a case of tendonitis in my right shoulder resulted in my doctor ordering me to complete eight weeks of physical therapy before he would refer me to an orthopedic specialist. The therapist worked my shoulder hard and gave me stretches and other exercises to do at home. After several weeks, my arm actually felt worse, and I insisted on seeing the orthopedist (and would have paid for the visit myself if necessary), who diagnosed tendonitis and told me that all I needed was to rest my arm. The physical therapy was actually contraindicated for my injury and was making the situation worse instead of better. I was fortunate that two weeks of simply wearing a sling after work ended the entire ordeal and that the physical therapy had not made the situation significantly more serious.

Some physicians might be too passive for your taste, while others are overly aggressive. Remember that you are the ultimate expert on your own body and only you know, simply from living in your own skin day in and day out, what is normal for you. An aggressive doctor will consider something to be a symptom and insist on further investigation when you know full well that it is perfectly normal for you. Under these circumstances, it is acceptable to say "no" to treatment or tests that you feel are premature or unwarranted. On the other hand, your doctor may be more willing than you are to give a condition time to either develop definitive symptoms or possibly to resolve on its own. If your intuition makes you anxious and worried, insist on some initial diagnostic steps. Occasionally, the doctor is more willing than the patient is to "wait things out," and you may have to consult a specialist who doesn't appear to be feeling his way along.

The Patient Wants to Explore Other Treatment Options

A physician may feel strongly about his proposed treatment plan and may not present any other options to the patient or be agreeable to searching for other treatment choices. One physician may feel that immediate surgery is the only viable option while a second doctor may be willing to try a more conservative treatment. Since there are often several acceptable choices for a particular diagnosis, you need to work with a physician who is willing to treat you as an individual, evaluate your unique situation and include you in all decisions.

These days, there are more alternative therapy choices than ever. Some that are considered commonplace today were originally met with great skepticism by the medical community. One dramatic example is the story of children with epilepsy who have dozens of seizures a day that do not respond to conventional medications. A ketogenic diet, which was high fat and low carbohydrate, was first developed in the 1920s and used until the 1940s until "newer, better" medications came along. It is highly effective in reducing seizures in some of these children. The problem, in the mid-1990s, was that not many people knew about it since it was out of favor. Then, in 1994, Dateline, ran a story on the diet, and in 1997 a made-for-TV movie starring Meryl Streep was shown, both of which brought the topic to the public's attention. Parents of children who had uncontrolled seizures immediately insisted on trying it. The diet is not a magic cure for everyone who tries it but it does work for some children. Imagine going through years of hopelessness because your doctor had either never heard of an option or knew of it but considered it unproven junk medicine and not worth mentioning when, in fact, it was the only solution that had any chance of success for you.

You should not feel pressured or coerced into accepting a treatment plan as the only option because it rarely is. Simply walking into another hospital across town could lead to a workable approach for a condition that was presented to you as hopeless. If your physician is not supportive of adjunctive therapies such as nutritional supplements or homeopathic remedies, and you think they could be of benefit, pursue these avenues on your own or look for a provider who will be more open to new approaches. Many patients have experienced unexpected recoveries or have improved dramatically in ways that defied all conventional expectations and could not be attributed to modern medicine. Physicians should be open to their patients trying alternative treatments including Eastern therapies, relaxation techniques, visualization, music therapy, or even aromatherapy, which have all been shown to have benefits for some patients. A doctor who discounts the value of other therapies simply because he didn't learn about them in medical school may be worth side-stepping for someone more open-minded.

Medicine evolves and changes and new therapies that start out as cutting edge often become commonplace, but a great number of patients freely chose them *before* they were generally accepted because the only other choice was unpalatable. It wasn't so long ago that a lumpectomy and radiation as an alternative to mastectomy was considered controversial. Progressive surgeons and oncologists started to wonder if every therapy for breast cancer had to be so disfiguring and invasive. "Is it really necessary to keep doing it this way just because that is the way it's always been done?" they wanted to know. The mainstream medical community felt comfortable with the more aggressive treatment because, after all, losing a breast seemed like a small price to pay for a cure. But for some women, it was not a small price at all. They were hungry for the opportunity to try something new and were willing to live with the consequences if it ultimately turned out to be less successful than mastectomy.

Think of the pioneer spirit of patients who allowed their heart surgeons to place stents in their arteries instead of having invasive cardiac surgeries. Patients with mental illness often choose psychotherapy as an alternative to taking medications that leave them feeling inhuman and profoundly apathetic. Women who are prone to chronic bladder infections were ecstatic to try drinking cranberry juice to lower their urine pH instead of taking antibiotics on and off for months at a time, which increased their odds of developing antibiotic resistance. Simply put, many people are willing to assume some risk in order to avoid more invasive procedures or prolonged drug regimens, and their experiences provide the data that validates the efficacy of new therapies.

The Prescribed Treatment is Simply Not Working for the Patient

If an individual is not responding to treatment, there are a number of possible explanations for it:

1. The original diagnosis isn't correct and has to be re-evaluated to rule out the possibility that that is why the treatment isn't effective. This has been covered above.

2. The original treatment plan is not proving as successful as hoped and, if there is no other alternative to explore, needs to be modified in some way to meet an individual patient's needs.

3. The patient wants to continue some form of treatment in an abbreviated form for quality of life issues. She wants another plan, not because she expects a cure, but simply to minimize symptoms or extend life. The story of one patient I interviewed for this book perfectly illustrates the last point. She had lung cancer, which had spread to her lymph nodes—a very bad sign. Her own doctor had placed her on chemotherapy, but it was not slowing the growth of a large mass under her right arm, which was extremely painful and was making her dependent on large doses of narcotic pain medications. Repeatedly, Mrs. R. asked her oncologist to try radiation, only to be told that it would not cure her. On her own, this patient consulted a radiologist, who explained that, while radiation wouldn't actually cure her cancer, it would undoubtedly shrink the mass under her arm, allowing her to sleep at night and to use less pain medication. Mrs. R. proceeded with the radiation, and it did afford her a much better quality of life, even if only for a few months.

4. The patient has lifestyle considerations or personal fears that make the treatment incompatible. She may be self-employed and need a plan that will allow her to work as many hours a week as possible. She may be too debilitated to drive long distances and require a hospital or treatment center closer to home. She could be living on a fixed income and not be able to pay for more elaborate care. Or she could have childcare issues and find it unworkable to be away from home for long periods of time. A patient who is deathly afraid of needles or who is claustrophobic may put off or even cancel having blood draws or MRI scans. Many institutions now have "open" scanning machines and there is a medication called EMLA that can be placed on the skin prior to drawing blood to numb the skin. But your doctor won't be able to use these new

options if he doesn't know about your needs up front. In all of these cases, input and honesty from the patient right from the beginning will give the plan the greatest chance of being set up to meet his individual needs.

5. An issue that is looming large as a problem in America is that some treatment plans include costly medications, especially newly approved drugs that are financially inaccessible to some patients. Everyone wishes access to the best drugs, but patients have to be realistic about their ability to pay for them. We have all heard the horror stories of aging patients with limited resources who've had to choose between medications and food. Others have resorted to cutting their medications in half or taking them on a sporadic schedule because that is the only way they can afford them. Be honest about your circumstances, and let your physician know if the cost of drugs will interfere with using the medication exactly as prescribed. Ask your physicians if they can provide medication samples for you to try in order to assess efficacy before you invest in expensive prescriptions that may not work. You should find out if there is a generic brand that is more affordable, and ask your doctor to contact the drug company to see if it has an access program for patients with limited financial resources. Even though patients often don't know about them, most of the major drug companies have "patient assistance programs" to make their drugs accessible to patients who cannot afford to pay for them. You may want to contact the drug company yourself via the Internet and request the appropriate form to save time. One of the nation's largest drug companies, Pfizer, has established a discount plan for uninsured and low-income Americans. For more information, call 866-706-2400. Websites to check are www.rxhope.com 732-507-7270, Partnership for Patient Assistance at www.pparx.org at 1-888-477-2669 or www.patientadvocate.org at 1-800-532-5274 which offers a patient assistance program to help pay co-payments on medications—www.copays.org at 1-866-512-3861.

6. The patient doesn't want to use prescription drugs, even when prescribed. This group represents a growing segment of the population who wishes to try an herbal or holistic approach. In my own dental practice, I deal with this fairly regularly. It is frustrating for everyone involved because the healthcare provider believes everything is going well and is dismayed to find out that the prescription hasn't been filled. The patient isn't being honest with his doctor about his intentions or his personal philosophy. He actually wants to minimize or even eliminate medication from his treatment, but isn't being up front with the one in charge of his care. Sometimes my patients actually fill the prescription, and then they don't take it or take it for a short time. I will get a call telling me they're still in pain or have other symptoms, and I can't understand why until they tell me what's been going on. Sometimes I find out they're having adverse effects to the medication and just stopped taking it, or that they have concerns about it and I can clear them up quickly. Addressing any issues up front keeps the communications channels open, and it saves a lot of time and trouble down the line.

7. Drug treatment can be considered "not working" if one medication is having an adverse interaction with another. Older patients are more likely to be on multiple drug regimens, prescribed by more than one doctor. Any one of these medications might be well tolerated individually, but in combination they cause devastating side effects. Physicians are not pharmacists, and they aren't mind readers. They need to hear about all of your medications, even over-the-counter or herbal drugs, and to find out who prescribed them in case a consultation is necessary. (Keep an updated medication list in your wallet so that physicians' offices can make a copy of it—it will save time and guarantee that nothing will be missed.) Patients should confer with their pharmacist and make sure that all their medications are compatible with the others, not just rely on their physician to predict every potential problem

involved in combining drug therapies. Large chain pharmacies utilize computerized information to alert pharmacists to drug interactions, so it helps to fill prescriptions at the same pharmacy so there is one record of all your medications. This increases the odds that the pharmacy's computer will catch a drug interaction. In addition, even if you place your medications into a weekly or monthly dispenser to remind yourself to take them, always keep the original bottle handy. This will allow any caregivers, family members or emergency personnel to have immediate access to information about your medications and their exact dosages.

8. A drug might present an unpleasant effect of its own that leads the patient to abandon therapy. In my own practice, I regularly see patients, who are prescribed blood pressure medications or antidepressants by their physician, develop extremely dry mouths. Unfortunately, this common side effect was never mentioned in the doctor's office, and the patient is doomed to suffer silently. To compensate for the lack of saliva, patients will often suck on hard candy, which can lead fairly quickly to rampant tooth decay. Imagine what that does to the patient's blood pressure or mental state: he may now need thousands of dollars of expensive dental work, he could even lose a few teeth, and he could be in pain and not able to chew very well. And all the problems could have been avoided if the patient knew that a dry mouth is a risk factor for tooth decay and had been instructed to see her dentist immediately, since there are many preventive strategies dentists have at their disposal. Perhaps a different blood pressure drug can be substituted, or at the very least, the patient's dentist can provide cavity prevention therapies and more frequent examinations to check for tooth decay.

Other kinds of drugs also have undesirable side effects. Psychotropic drugs, for instance, are often discontinued by patients because they make them feel zombie-like, sleepy or prone to weight gain. Medications that cause diarrhea, constipation or loss of appetite can become so problematic to manage that patients make the decision on their own to stop using them. Read the handout from the pharmacy and find out the most likely side effects. Patients tell me that they don't read the information from the pharmacy because it lists so many potential side effects that it causes them to imagine that they will have each and every one of them! Pay closest attention to the ones at the top of the list since they are considered the most common. If constipation, for example, is a likely side effect, don't wait more than a couple of days without a bowel movement before you consult your doctor about taking appropriate measures. Adding some fiber to your diet or an over-the-counter stool softener pill can make the difference between staying on a needed drug or stopping it in frustration.

Whatever the cause is for the inappropriateness of your treatment plan, the key before even seeking an opinion from another physician is to be honest with the one you have. If you aren't comfortable speaking up yourself, let an advocate do it for you. Don't, for instance, let your doctor keep handing you prescriptions you can't afford. Don't make up excuses for not coming into the doctor's office for a shot without disclosing that you're scared. There could be another way. In fact, don't let down your end of the responsibility and put your health at risk because you are worried, guilty, broke, burdened, or uncomfortable about your physician's prescribed course of action. Just as you want your doctor to be honest with you, you must also be honest with him. A relationship marred by deceit or lack of honesty could prove harmful to you. And don't wait to express your concerns. Treatment, especially for a serious illness, is a weighty matter. Putting the matter off can cause you to shift gears in your treatment mid-stream, which will be frustrating for you and cause unnecessary difficulty for doctors and staff.

It is vital for the public to know that clinical trials or experimental treatments may be appropriate for patients whose condition is not responding to traditional therapies. If your physician isn't supportive of this alternative, or he doesn't seem willing to expend the effort to help look for a clinical trial for your condition, it might be a reason to obtain another opinion. Naturally, physicians cannot be aware of every single new treatment modality or clinical trial available, but they should be receptive to the concept and be willing to assist patients in exploring these options. A patient might want to volunteer to participate in medical research to have access to investigational drugs or treatments not yet available to the general public. However, there is no guarantee of admission to a study. The criteria for entering such research studies are usually very specific and/or restrictive, and it may not even be an option until all other traditional treatment modalities have failed. There may also be fees associated with the program that are not covered by the patient's health insurance. Patients can investigate research studies or clinical studies by contacting the following groups:

www.centerwatch.com (617) 856-5900. Every time a new clinical trial is announced that relates to the patient's diagnosis, Centerwatch will send email alerts to those who register. This site also has a valuable resources guide.

www.clinicaltrials.gov The National Institutes of Health maintains a database for clinical trials.

www.ucsf.edu/research/clinicaltrials This site lists all of San Francisco's University of California trials, and includes contact information.

www.cancer.gov National Cancer Institute Clinical Trials Database.

www.cancertrials.stanford.edu Stanford University Medical Center can also be contacted at (650)-498-7061.

www.cancercenter.standord.edu/clinicaltrials/search (650) 498-7061.

The Patient Doesn't Feel that He or She is Part of the Team

The amount and the quality of the communication between the doctor and the patient (or the patient's family) are vital components of a proactive approach to medical care. Some doctors, of course, are more adept than others at communicating effectively. Patients who genuinely want to be informed and to function as a contributing member of their own medical team will be frustrated if:

1. Their doctors' communication skills are poor.

2. Their doctors' management of their case seems deficient in any area and they aren't telling them what's going on.

3. They have side effects that are not being managed properly, and no one seems to care. Nausea, immune function, and pain management are areas of treatment that often need either a customized approach or a referral to a specialist. In modern medicine, patients not only need a physician who can treat the disease itself, but can also control the side effects of treatment.

Since the amount and quality of communication between you and your doctor are vital to your care, don't underestimate the importance of convincing him to keep you in the loop. A key component of this is the level of your physician's communication skills. This goes for other members of your medical team, too. Nurses, medical assistants, physical therapists and nutritionists all need to talk to you in accessible language, keep you informed and make sure you're in agreement with their plan.

You have a certain responsibility here also. Are you taking it upon yourself to be a full member of the team? Have you made it perfectly clear how important it is to be involved? Have you expressed the kind of information you want made available to you? You need to state that your goal is to be a full participant in your care, not to convey the message, "You're the doctor. I'm just the patient. You just do whatever you think is best." You must also assume responsibility for keeping the lines of communication open and for taking part in decisions. Make it clear that you want to be updated regularly on your treatment plan so that you always know what is coming up next. If you have a doctor who seems completely unnerved, and perhaps even resentful, by this level of information sharing, then it is time for a switch. There is nothing wrong in telling a physician "We just don't seem to be a good match."

Whenever you feel that you are in the dark about your progress, you must say so. If you find yourself continually surprised by a test, a doctor's visit, a blood sample, or an x-ray, that is a clear sign you're not being treated as a full member of the team. If you have a test or a procedure and no one tells you the results, you're not a full-fledged member. Even receiving an oral message about the results isn't always the best idea. I recommend that you obtain copies of the written reports from all blood tests, scans, x-rays or pathology results, and keep them in a binder for easy reference. The medical office should be happy to do this for you. If you have left the hospital or the doctor's office and you don't have a fax machine at home, provide them with a self-addressed, stamped envelope as a courtesy.

As an informed member of the team, you will be able to evaluate the overall effectiveness of the group as a whole. Are the other members of the team communicating and consulting with each other? For example, your doctor needs to know how your physical therapy is progressing, all the medications prescribed by other physicians, the results of tests ordered by specialists, and if you are following the recommendations of a nutritionist or dietician. Your doctor should be staying informed via phone calls or written reports from the other providers. Either way, there should be a detailed notation in your chart about every aspect of your care, including the ones that don't happen in the doctor's office. Your chart, which functions as the owner's manual for your body, should be organized efficiently to allow your doctor to have all the pertinent information literally at his fingertips. Ask if the physical therapist or cardiologist has been keeping your doctor updated about your progress. A quick run-down from you, the patient, is not a substitute so ask your other providers to provide regular progress notes to your physician.

Members of a team may strive to work toward a shared, common goal, but that doesn't mean that they always agree on the best way to get there. If one person on the team tells you one thing and someone else contradicts it, first be concerned that they have not conferred with each other. Verify that everyone has spoken to each other face to face or through a personal phone call, not just via voice mail or through assistants. Second, be attuned to any undertones of disagreement, because it may mean that some aspect of your treatment is in question and there has been no consensus on the correct course of action. Insist that you be informed if there is a disagreement, told what it is concerning, understand the rationale behind the different approaches, and are vocal about your needs and opinions. Any member of the team who is hindering progress, or who doesn't respect your right to be informed, can always be replaced.

The Doctor has a Style of Operating and Making Decisions that Doesn't Mesh with the Patient's

Never underestimate the benefit of having a doctor whose personality, style of operating, and way of making decisions are aligned with your own. Not only do you have to get to know the doctor, she has to get to know you and to understand your family situation and its unique circumstances. Patients often express surprise at their "luck" in finding that particular chemistry, but this doesn't have to be left to chance.

In the old days, compassion, respect, comfort, trust and support were the cornerstones of the medical profession. When there was a closer one-on-one relationship with the physician, it wasn't unusual for patients to feel understood and taken care of. You can create that for yourself if you are more vocal about your fears, needs, desires and hopes. You might need a great deal more reassurance than you are asking for. Desperately ill patients are usually much more terrified of feeling abandoned by the medical system, having their doctor give up on them, or of not having their pain controlled than they are of actually dying.

This said, your doctor does not have to be someone you would choose as a best friend; you're not required to have each other over for dinner on Saturday night. It simply means that your physician must have an approach and a demeanor that allow you to work in tandem with her toward a common goal, and that you are able to sustain this satisfactory relationship over an extended period of time, if necessary. Be realistic here, since feelings of frustration, anger and disillusionment often amplify as you work your way through a challenging treatment plan. A good working relationship doesn't mean that there are never disagreements, but it does mean that conflict can always be resolved to your satisfaction.

When thinking about personality and style, it is important to know how "hands-on" you would like your doctor to be in your care. If you want a physician who is involved in all the details, you will never be satisfied with one who manages your treatment plan from a distance or from behind a closed door. You might not want one who relies too heavily on nurses, assistants, or even other doctors to treat you. And you will certainly ask that he be available for consultation and to answer your questions at all visits or at in-office chemotherapy appointments.

Any patient who is consistently dissatisfied with the accessibility level of his physician should consider seeking the advice, and possibly, the care of another doctor. If your doctor is part of a larger group practice, you may not be entitled to see a single provider on every visit; you may be expected to see whichever doctor is available. Ask right up front if you will be able to see the doctor of your choice at every visit. This could require that you schedule on certain days or times, and this is not an unreasonable request. Even if you start with one doctor in the practice, you might find another who is preferable, so ask if patients are allowed to switch to other doctors. You will also want to find out whom you will be directed to after hours if there is an urgent situation. Sometimes patients are managed by a doctor they've never met and one who isn't even a member of that practice right in the middle of an emergency. Naturally this could be very disconcerting, so find out in advance if there are going to be any surprises.

Another aspect of a doctor's style is his lifestyle. Does your doctor travel extensively to conferences to give lectures to other physicians, thereby rendering him inaccessible to you on a regular basis? The travel schedule of your doctor may be counterproductive to the continuity of your care, even if it is beneficial for his career advancement. When you first see the doctor, ask how often he is away from his practice.

Yet another aspect of style you need to inquire into is that of the office itself. How is it managed? When you call, can you talk to an actual person, or will you be rerouted endlessly through a series of recorded messages? In the end, do you end up having to press a dozen buttons only to leave a message on a machine? And how quickly are your calls returned? If you feel ill and have a question about a symptom, it will not work for you if the office doesn't call you back until a week later — that will cause far too many sleepless nights. When you have to request refills on a prescription with a message on the office's voicemail, do they phone it in right away or do you have to keep calling them back, asking when the doctor will get around to it? For some offices, over-scheduling is a routine part of the practice, and you might feel more comfortable, and receive more attentive care, at a different office.

It is a fact of human interaction that everyone is off his or her mark occasionally. No physician or medical practice is absolutely perfect, but the way they operate should be consistently up to par since a good doctor-patient relationship plays such a significant role in successful medical care.

The Patient Has a Problem with the Doctor's Level of Experience, Competence or Ethics

Too many people are uneasy about inquiring into a physician's skills and/or experience. You should know that it is never inappropriate to ask how many patients with your condition your doctor has treated. Or to ask if he is a specialist. Or to find out if he is board-certified. (To become board-certified, physicians must take certification exams and meet continuing education requirements.)

If you find yourself with a doctor who just doesn't seem knowledgeable about your condition, how can you feel confident remaining in his care? The same is true if he is not competent or confident, if he is nervous or unsure. And what if he doesn't seem to hold himself to a particularly high code of ethical standards? Perhaps his manner is too familiar or you notice that he is billing out for extended office visits even after a short "quick check" appointment. Your instincts and gut impressions can be trusted to tell you when any of these conditions are present. You may not be absolutely certain, but it shouldn't keep you from inquiring into it.

A shocking event at a medical center in California illustrates the importance of challenging advice that seems questionable, even if it comes from a respected physician. A respected cardiologist, who was the Director of Cardiology at the center, saw a patient with a family history of heart disease for a treadmill test. After the test, the doctor ordered a cardiac catheterization test. After catheterization, the doctor told the patient, who was, by the way, completely asymptomatic, that he needed bypass surgery immediately. The surprised patient might have followed the advice, but a friend persuaded him to seek a second opinion first. The new tests revealed no coronary artery disease. A subsequent inquiry revealed that dozens of other patients were frightened or coerced into having procedures that did not appear to be necessary. While a single case could have been attributed to an error in the testing procedure, the sheer number of patients who were misdiagnosed by this cardiologist stood out. Another patient was told that he was having a heart attack right at the moment he was speaking to the doctor and that he would die without immediate surgery. Another patient, a father of three, was informed that his minor chest pains were from a clogged artery, and if he didn't have surgery right away, his chance of survival was zero. Yet another patient was recovering from an appendectomy when the cardiologist appeared at his bedside and told him he was ordering an angiogram to check his heart. Naturally, the patient was bewildered that a cardiologist showed up at all. He sensed that something was amiss, but couldn't bring himself to say no to the test. He was even more shocked when the doctor later told him he had a heart problem referred to as the "widow maker." In all of these cases, further examination revealed that none of these diagnoses were true, and the world only found out about it when *60 Minutes* aired a report on the story.

Most of the above patients, like many patients who have placed themselves in a doctor's care, were extremely reluctant to distrust their doctor's advice, even though his intuition told them something was wrong. In the above cases, the physician was investigated and stopped practicing medicine. Fortunately this is rare, and a great majority of doctors are acting in the best interest of their patients. However, physicians are human. If they are experiencing personal problems of their own, it could affect the level of care they provide. Doctors are as likely as the rest of us to be stricken by financial problems, illness, substance abuse, or family crises. If your physician ever seems overwhelmed, distracted or unprepared, or if he has done something that even appears unethical, pay attention to your gut feeling and take the initiative to seek another opinion. Remember that only a small number of medical conditions require intervention so instantaneous that the patient doesn't have time to consult with another physician. It is a rare event that a patient has to make a sudden decision about her medical treatment.

There is a Difference in Philosophy About Whether to Continue Treatment or to End it

Just as it is important to share a similar style, so, too, it matters if you and your doctor have similar philosophies about treatment–when to continue it and when to end it. In my personal situation, my husband and I had a shared goal of wanting to support our daughter's decision about whether her quality of life merited continued treatment. Even when we all knew that a cure was no longer possible, Kate's indomitable spirit gave her a tremendous will to carry on. We could not discount or ignore it. For her, there was never any other option than to fight every step of the way.

Yet her oncologist, who had been treating her since she was five months old, unilaterally decided to stop her modified chemotherapy because of the increased risk of infection and the overwhelming odds that the cancer would recur anyway. We knew that Kate had already had several hospital-acquired infections, but she had recovered. The consequence of discontinuing chemo would be that the cancer, which was now gone from her body, would quickly return to her bones. Kate wanted to continue her treatment, in spite of the risks, but the oncologist was only willing to offer "plenty of morphine to keep her comfortable," and no treatment. We agreed with Kate and not the doctor. Allowing her to fight for her life had to be better than giving her up to an agonizing death from metastatic bone cancer.

Our trusted oncologist could not be swayed, so we obtained opinions from two other doctors, who both agreed to continue her chemo on a modified basis to suit her changing health needs. Even though the original oncologist was right–Kate succumbed to her disease–we ultimately chose to go with a physician who shared our philosophy on healthcare and end-of-life treatment. For a nine-year-old girl, 19 months is a long time, and we were able to give her a wonderful life during that period. We have never regretted our decision to let her lead the way in her own treatment.

Of course, patients and their families are not always right and must consider a decision to depart from doctor's orders very, very carefully. However, if the alternative treatment they seek is not reckless, if it has been working so far or has worked for others, and if the family is prepared to live with the consequences, then I feel that there are few valid reasons a doctor can offer to go against their wishes. I question the value of doctors making unilateral decisions just because they think they know better or have seen others with your condition fare poorly with the kind of decision you wish to make regarding your treatment. Life is unpredictable, and people do make seemingly miraculous recoveries all the time. They make extraordinary progress in ways that cannot be explained by modern medical wisdom. If you aren't given the opportunity to try, you will never know if you will be among the lucky.

Not every decision about whether to continue treatment involves terminal patients, a diagnosis of cancer or some other life-threatening disease. Certain kinds of treatment for other maladies are favored by some and looked down on by others. Estrogen replacement therapy is a case in point. Even though the medical community is more reluctant to offer it now because of recent research findings that are unfavorable, many women want to continue ERT anyway because of quality-of-life issues. For them, nothing else reduces hot flashes, migraines and any of the other symptoms the way ERT does. The side effects of menopause are so life-altering that it may be appropriate for these women to assume the risk of short-term hormone replacement.

Another example is hip replacement surgery. I have interviewed patients in their late 30s, a young age for such a problem, who were candidates for total hip replacement, but their surgeons were reluctant to do it. They advised postponing surgery indefinitely because of their age. The patients, however, were tired of putting up with limping, being in chronic pain, losing sleep and endlessly restricting their activities. They wanted to go ahead with the operation, even though they knew the effects of the procedure wouldn't last forever and that they would most likely have to go under the knife again.

On the other side of the spectrum are the patients who do not want to be treated at all. Because of risks, side effects, stress, the ordeal of therapy, or money worries, they want to end their treatment, or at least to minimize it considerably. A doctor could recommend surgery to a patient with a shoulder injury, but the person would rather live with the pain than go through an invasive procedure. Patients who have had several shoulder surgeries just to remove scar tissue have been known to stop the process and just deal with the problem in other ways. I recently spoke to a woman who had ovarian cysts that necessitated the removal of her ovaries. But the surgeon recommended removing her uterus as well "just to be safe," even though there was no uterine pathology or family history of such problems. Some women might have gone along with the plan, but this patient decided that as long as her uterus was all right, she wanted it left intact. The surgeon persisted, though, strongly advising her to have a total hysterectomy because she "might develop uterine cancer later." This was not a convincing argument to this individual who saw no reason to have an organ taken out of her body that was perfectly healthy. A majority of women go through their entire lives with their uterus intact, and if cancer was to be detected down the road, she was willing to accept the consequences.

Of course, none of these people made their decisions lightly. Before you decide to modify or stop any treatment, serious thought must be given. Patients can make hasty decisions because they are misinformed about consequences. Case in point is the large numbers of people every year who are prescribed antibiotic drugs, choose to go off the prescription early because they "feel better now." They fail to realize that they are putting themselves at risk for an even more potent infection that could now be resistant to the medication, and ought to listen to their doctors. And it is imperative that patients who choose to forego invasive medical intervention sign a Do Not Resuscitate order (DNR) and provide copies to their loved ones and to the hospital. A signed DNR should be readily visible in your home because if paramedics rush through the door and your advocate cannot find the signed form, you will be given heroic life-saving measures. Patients are sometimes afraid to sign these orders because they fear that they will be denied pain medication or oxygen, but this is not the case. Palliative, or comfort measures, are not included in DNR's. If it causes you concern, be sure to add a sentence or two on the document specifically stating that you want to be kept comfortable at all times and that you are NOT refusing oxygen, pain control or other palliative measures.

The decision to continue, modify or end treatment is a delicate balancing act between risk assessment and the potential benefits. Never make such a choice unless you have taken the time to be informed about your condition and your options and made every effort to partner with a physician who is respectful of your individual preferences and tolerances.

The Patient's Intuition is Telling Her That Something isn't Right

Far too often, patients dismiss their intuitive feelings because they have no medical experience or training. "Who am I to question someone who has gone to medical school?" Sometimes, however, a patient's common sense or gut feeling can rival years of formal training and education. In his book, *The Gift of Fear,* author Gavin de Becker says that our instincts should never be ignored in any life event, including medical emergencies. De Becker is a leading safety expert who implores the public to both acknowledge and act on the "survival signals" that alert human beings to danger. Survival strategies revolve around the innate gut feelings we all have that signal us about the possibility of danger. We are all familiar with the fight-or-flight response, in which subtle and imperceptible signals guide our split-second decisions. This is a natural gift the same way that intuition is. When any of my patients feel intimidated or uncomfortable with a healthcare provider, I routinely advise them to act on it and make a change. I tell them to keep searching until they find a relationship that fosters peace of mind.

This is not to undermine the value of pure knowledge or to relieve anyone of the responsibility to be informed. I am only saying that intuition is also a vital component of healthcare safety. Patients with deep misgivings about their physician, diagnosis, or treatment plan—even if they cannot articulate what is wrong—should not hesitate to seek another opinion. I have never heard of a situation in which there was only one doctor on the entire planet who could treat a particular patient, so don't settle for a relationship with someone when your gut instinct is warning you away.

Second Opinion Sources

1. Your own doctor. Ask him or her for a referral to a physician outside their practice. If he is affiliated with a hospital, ask for a name outside that hospital. But be careful here. Whoever he refers you to might be a colleague, and colleagues are notorious for not wanting to contradict each other. Your doctor may also have a propensity to associate with physicians who take the same approach he does.

2. Nurses or other healthcare professionals you may know or that your friends or family members may be acquainted with. Even if nurses are unwilling to share their misgivings about a certain physician, they are usually willing to discreetly steer you in the right direction.

3. Referral services provided by hospitals, support groups or the local medical society.

4. Local or national resource organizations such as the American Cancer Society, the National Cancer Institute, and the American Heart Association.

5. Family members or friends who have had a positive experience with a particular physician and believe the recommendation to be appropriate.

6. Your health insurance company.

7. Names from Internet searches. Online searches can provide the names and contact information for physicians who are the recognized experts in their field. You can also conduct a search for doctors who have published articles or conducted research on your condition.

8. Major medical centers, regional cancer centers, or university hospitals.

9. www.blochcancer.org provides a list of multi-disciplinary second opinion institutions.

Resources for Second Opinions on Pathology Specimens

www.findcancerexperts.com matches patients with expert pathologists and provides contact information and instructions for obtaining and sending pathology specimens.

www.Mdexpert.com provides second opinions specifically for cancer diagnoses.

www.pathserv.com or contact their toll free number at (877) 612-2085.

www.bostwicklaboratories.com or Bostwick@bostwicklaboratories.com

Now That You've Decided . . .

Once you have chosen a physician for a second opinion, make sure you are honest and open when discussing your plans with your original doctor. Just because you're going to consult with someone else, it doesn't mean he jumps off the radar screen. First of all, he will need to send information to the consulting physician, and second, you could decide that you want to be treated by him after all. So don't burn any bridges.

Whenever you seek a second opinion, you're not erasing the past. You don't just visit another office across town and start completely over. The consulting physician has to see what has happened up until this point. She needs your hospital and/or office medical records, copies of all radiology tests (CT, MRI, bone scans, chest x-rays, etc.), original pathology slides, copies of reports from any recent blood studies, and copies of the written reports from any diagnostic testing. Since consulting physicians do not rely solely on written reports, the actual x-rays or scans are also necessary.

After the new doctor receives all pertinent information, be prepared for her to order additional tests or to request that existing studies be repeated. Different physicians and hospitals require their own confirmation of a diagnosis or test result, and they might not proceed with the data from another provider or institution.

This process isn't always an easy ride for the patient. You have to realize that the information and recommendations from another medical opinion will not necessarily put you at ease, but could leave you feeling stressed and confused. Sometimes, three different physicians will offer three different plans of action for the same diagnosis; the reason is that there are almost always several acceptable approaches to the same problem. It will help you make a decision if you understand the reasoning and logic behind their choices and comprehend how they arrived at their conclusions. The first question you should ask is, "Why do you feel that this is the appropriate treatment for my condition and for me as an individual?"

Doing the above will ensure that a flawed decision-making process did not determine your treatment plan, or that the plan wasn't based on personal preference and habit instead of scientific research and current standard of care criteria. A little lesson in history will put this into perspective: Years after procedures such as lumpectomies and angioplasty became widely accepted, many doctors went right on advising patients to have mastectomies and bypass surgery instead. That is what these physicians were used to, and that is what they recommended, even though the newer treatments were less invasive, less costly and easier to recover from. Nowadays, lumpectomies, where appropriate, routinely lessen physical and emotional trauma, reduce the need for invasive reconstructive surgery and leave patients with their self-esteem intact. Press your doctor to tell you what all the options are for your condition. Ask if she is aware of recent research or updated medical advice for your illness. If you have taken the time to research your diagnosis yourself, your inquiries will be more specific and informed. This, of course, underscores the need for patients to gather their own information. It will prepare them for discussions with their physicians that will allow them to plan treatment in a meaningful way.

Play Your Part

I cannot stress enough how important it is to take the time to establish a relationship with your primary care physician before you are diagnosed with a serious illness. Not only will he be making life-and-death decisions about you, but he is often the gatekeeper for a referral to a specialist and he plays a major role in the second opinion process. You must also be informed about the details of your insurance coverage and how it applies to second opinions. If you have to spend precious time in the middle of a health crisis trying to establish an instant relationship with your physician, it will place you at a real disadvantage. You also don't want to find yourself in the position of going through a crash course in the intricacies of your medical plan rather than spending your time researching the best medical options for your condition.

I recommend obtaining an updated patient handbook from your insurance company. These booklets contain general information about covered benefits, and they are a good starting point for searching out further facts. Customer service representatives at the insurance company can answer some questions, but don't rely on their statements as a guarantee that any service you ask for will be covered under your plan. For any special services that you require, obtain authorization in advance, or you might have to pay out of your own pocket. If you need a second opinion (or even a third opinion) and the insurance company is dragging its heels, be prepared to pay for it yourself. You may be able to seek reimbursement later. Whatever the insurance company's position is, too much is on the line to overlook this potentially life-saving option.

Chapter Six

When Reality Does Not Meet Your Expectations

Communicating Your Concerns and Complaints

Fortunately, most hospital stays are brief, peaceful and uneventful; medical treatment proceeds as planned, outcomes are successful, and patients leave the hospital healthier than when they came in. But for a growing number of patients, hospitalization creates more problems than it solves. Patients return home after experiencing doubts, concerns, and life-threatening complications. They might be dissatisfied with their diagnosis, treatment plan, or recovery recommendations, and often the origin of their doubts and conflicts can be attributed to a simple lack of communication or a misunderstanding between them and their healthcare providers.

We have all heard media reports about the dangers that arise from a serious breach in the communication process. The most notorious are the cases where one patient is mistaken for another. The unfortunate patient then goes on to have an operation he doesn't need at all, and the one who does need it goes untreated. Those are the TV-worthy stories. What patients don't hear about as often is the high price they pay for the incessant, seemingly "harmless glitches" that, in reality, can set the stage for a breakdown in communication and the resulting endless cavalcade of errors. A recent situation involving my aunt is a perfect example of how easy it is for a series of crossed signals to impact a hospital stay in a negative way.

While hospitalized for hernia surgery, my Aunt Rose felt that she was having excessive pain, but as soon as the new shift nurse entered her room, she announced, "You're doing great. You haven't even used much pain medicine," and proceeded to take vital signs. My aunt, being tired and somewhat dazed having just emerged from her anesthesia, had heard the nurse state emphatically that she was doing well, and she hesitated to disagree with her. What was particularly confusing was that she *had* been pushing the button to release medication frequently, yet the nurse insisted she wasn't using "much." By the time it occurred to her to say something, the nurse had already left the room. Rose never realized that the nurse could be mistaken, so she just thought that she was being hypersensitive about the pain. And so she suffered in silence, assuming that the nurse could assess her condition better than she could herself.

Hours later, my aunt's daughter-in-law came to visit; Rose informed her of the earlier conversation with the nurse. The young woman looked at the pump and noticed that the numbers were lit up but not changing when Rose self-administered a dose, which meant that her mother-in-law needed, and failed to get, medication simply because the pump was not delivering it. The nurse was summoned and quickly discovered that the machine was indeed plugged in, but that it had not been reset after Rose left the recovery room.

Three things contributed to this situation:

1. My aunt did not communicate what she knew to be true. She was, in fact, in pain. If Rose had simply said, "I might seem like I'm doing OK, but actually I'm not," it would have alerted the nurse that further assessment was needed. Unfortunately, you cannot always count on medicated patients to speak up, which is why having an advocate stay with the patient is invaluable.

2. The nurse made erroneous assumptions about Rose's pain level without specifically asking her about it. The lesson here is for patients to speak up if their providers seem to be relying too heavily on machines or numeric values when they seem at odds with their personal experiences.

3. A "glitch" in hospital procedures allowed Rose to be transferred to another unit without the pump being checked and reset.

   When you observe even one glitch, you can probably assume that it has happened before and will happen again if somebody doesn't intervene and try to change it. After I asked Rose if she had issued a complaint or taken any action to prevent the problem from happening again, she seemed bewildered; surely her nurse had taken care of all that. I could understand that in my aunt's condition, just out of surgery and woozy from morphine, she might not want to take on the complaint process. But, her daughter-in-law was in the perfect position to ask the nurse to report the incident to the proper supervisor. As happened with my aunt, though, it never came to mind. Rose could also have initiated a complaint as soon as she felt well enough, or even via a phone call after she returned home.

After an incident like this, it may seem that no harm was done so it's fine to let it go, but we all have to become more altruistic about these occurrences. It is not enough to breathe a sigh of relief when you get home and say, "Well, that wasn't so bad. At least they didn't cut off the wrong leg or kill me." Think about it though: in many other situations, we think nothing of warning others about life's pitfalls. Consider the number of occasions that you take the time to spare friends and neighbors mere inconveniences, like telling them to put their garbage cans out on time, move their cars on street cleaning day, or avoid certain roads because of traffic congestion. Think how important it is to you to be sure that any danger you have identified or lived through is one that you can spare your loved ones. Somehow in hospital situations we have not cultivated this same mindset.

To make effective complaints, you have to first know what's gone wrong, and there are basically two ways for you to find out. One is that you experience an adverse event personally and you have an idea what is causing it. Or, two, someone who works at the hospital is honest enough to tell you something went wrong. All hospitals have their own internal administrative systems to deal with patient problems, but, of course, a patient must rely on a staff member to be told that there is a problem or figure out on her own that something is amiss. What you must realize is that whatever incident – big or small – that you are going through, it may be only the tip of the iceberg. The true extent of the problem could be far greater than you know. It could, in fact, be system-wide. Some hospitals are implementing policies to inform patients of errors or of iatrogenic injury (injury caused by doctors or medical treatment), but at this time *there is no comprehensive, universally applied federal law or regulation stating that every institution must inform patients when they have been the recipients of faulty medical treatment.* A few individual states have implemented mandatory error reporting laws, including Nevada, Florida, New Jersey, Vermont, Pennsylvania, Minnesota and California. Hopefully, these progressive states will inspire every state to do the same. Of course, the next step would be the establishment of one centralized entity to track the data, make comparisons, and act as a vehicle to immediately disseminate information about errors and risks.

As a result, for decades, patients have been kept in the dark about injuries caused by the very hospital they put their hope and faith in.

People might have an inkling when something is wrong because they are in excessive pain, their recovery is prolonged, or their infection won't go away. If a pair of forceps has been left in a patient's abdomen, she might not be aware of it until she finally sets off an airport metal detector at a later date. Don't laugh—this very situation actually happened in 2002. Even if the risk manager or hospital administrator is "looking into" their situation, patients cannot assume that the institution is motivated only by concern for the individual's welfare. Hospitals have been known to keep pertinent information away from patients to avoid trouble. Remember that they employ lawyers and other risk management personnel to handle potentially litigious patients. If you cause a stir, they might mount a defense, advise their staff on how to respond to your inquiries cautiously, and quietly review your medical record as a way of heading trouble off at the pass. I am not saying that the administration is "against you," but it certainly views you as someone they need to protect themselves against if it looks like you are voicing a complaint to people who can sanction them.

This method of doing business has left patients unaware of the many mechanisms in place, both inside and outside the hospital walls, to assist them when there is an unfortunate incident. The purpose of this book is to raise the average person's medical IQ so that he will be able to recognize a threat to his well being, to register an intelligent and effective complaint, and, ultimately, to head off potential problems before they occur - which is a win-win situation for everyone.

Upon admission to the hospital, information should be readily provided explaining how to contact the patient relations department or what to do if you experience a problem. When you register, be sure that the admitting office provides you with information about the hospital's system for dealing with concerns or complaints. If problems arise that are not resolved by dealing directly with your treating physician or your nurse, you need to be aware of the other individuals and agencies with the authority to intervene on your behalf.

The individuals and groups are:

1. Charge Nurses and Nurse Managers

2. Patient Relations Specialists/Patient Advocates/Ombudsman

3. Social Services

4. Infection Control Specialist

5. Department Heads/Service Heads

6. Hospital Administration

7. Medical Center Director/Chief Operating Officer (COO)

8. Hospital Licensing and Certification

9. The Joint Commission on Accreditation of Healthcare Organizations ("the Joint Commission")

10. Medical Boards

11. The Media

There is a hierarchy of sorts when deciding whom to take a complaint to. The logical starting point is always your nurse and treating physician. But if you cannot reach a solution that is both timely and acceptable, start working your way through the above list. The Charge Nurse or Patient Relations Specialist will be able to handle a large percentage of patient complaints. Social Services and Infection Control Specialists may be able to handle specific issues regarding communication glitches with your caregivers or investigate the source of your infection. The head of a particular hospital department or medical "service" needs to be consulted if you have an issue with your physician or his treatment plan that cannot be resolved by talking to your doctor directly. For serious complaints such as the occurrence of life-threatening complications, "systems errors," or care that seems truly negligent or substandard, the hospital administration and possibly the COO need to be contacted. Situations involving patient safety issues, potential violations of current medical standards of care, and physician misconduct can be reported to hospital licensing boards, medical boards or to the Joint Commission. The media is the last, yet often the most powerful, resource to resort to.

Charge Nurses and Nurse Managers

The Charge Nurse is the direct supervisor of every nurse in a particular area or "unit" of the hospital. The first person in charge of your care, and therefore the first one to contact if you experience a problem is your bedside nurse. However, if she is not available or doesn't seem capable of handling your situation, you need to contact the Charge Nurse, who works closely with all the staff members in the unit to ensure a comprehensive team approach. He or she should be happy to consult directly with patients. All major areas of the hospital that provide direct patient care, including Pediatrics, Intensive Care Units and Emergency Departments, are likely to have a nurse functioning in this administrative capacity. Some departments in the hospital may not have a Charge Nurse on-site, but each and every nurse reports to an immediate advisor, so you can easily find out whom to contact next by asking your nurse to have her supervisor talk to you.

Often the only time you will have contact with the Charge Nurse is if there is a problem. Call her if you feel that your bedside nurse seems too busy to attend to the alarms on monitors or to administer medications on time. The Charge Nurse can consult with you about staff members who seem too tired, who aren't washing their hands, or who are distracted or brusque. The Charge Nurse has the authority to alter the staff assignments to be sure that your nurse is completely capable of meeting your needs. It is not uncommon to encourage nurses to gain experience by assigning them to patients who are actually a little too challenging for their skill level. But, if your nurse truly seems to be struggling, a change may be in order.

Charge Nurses have a number of duties: they supervise nursing personnel, evaluate the quality of care, establish effective policies and procedures for the unit, help develop individual care plans based on each patient's unique needs, may even provide direct patient care, and troubleshoot all problems in the unit, including patient complaints. Their observations and decisions about which nurse is assigned to what patient and how they use their staff is going to impact your stay as much as anything else. Simply put, Charge Nurses help make hospital care more responsive to the needs of patients. As such, they are available to consult when patients and their families are dissatisfied in any way. A patient I interviewed relayed this story. After surgery, her nurse told her that the doctor had written orders for her to have intravenous pain medication every two hours, as needed. After many extra hours of being in pain, however, the patient asked to speak to the Charge Nurse, who then reviewed the orders and discovered that the physician had also written an order for oral pain medication to be administered if the patient wasn't completely comfortable. In short, she was entitled to more medication than she was getting. Speaking up to the right person and bringing in a fresh perspective turned the miserable situation around.

Any problem not within the expertise or authority of a Charge Nurse should be directed to the Nurse Manager. It is important to know that nursing supervisors such as Nurse Managers are *always* able to contact a "House Supervisor" or other on-call administrator. Situations that warrant this intervention? A major medical error has occurred causing a deterioration of the patient's condition, a patient has been injured in an accident in the hospital, a patient has not seen a physician in a timely manner and this is hindering his treatment plan, or a patient's pain level is intolerably high. Pain is now referred to as the fifth "vital sign," meaning that its continual assessment and control are necessary to evaluate a patient's progress and to aid in her recovery. Remember that expecting the Nurse Manager to contact the hospital administration is an option that should be reserved for a true emergency, one that cannot wait until regular business hours.

Patients usually have no idea that it's even possible to ask for assistance from nursing supervisors and that there is a hierarchy that the staff can turn to if a serious situation arises. Your first line of defense is always your nurse—you don't want to jump ahead in the line of command by demanding that senior administrators attend to minor issues. The one constant you can count on is the nursing staff, who remain one of the most accessible and dynamic resources for patients and their loved ones.

Patient Relations Specialists/ Patient Advocates/Ombudsman

Patient Relations Specialists or representatives run interference for the hospital administration in the day-to-day running of the institution and act as gatekeepers, deciding which problems need the administration's immediate attention. In short, they function as liaisons between patients and the system, striving to find answers and solutions to the questions, concerns, and grievances that are an inevitable part of hospitalization. They might encounter requests for extended visiting hours to accommodate the work schedules of your advocates, rooming-in issues, problems with hospital housekeeping or overall cleanliness, and treatment by staff members that is disrespectful or intimidating.

Patient relations representatives constantly evaluate the quality of their hospital's patient care services, facilitate communication between patients and providers, educate both patients and staff members, and advocate for patient's rights. You can contact them about specific hospital policies and procedures, to help mediate any disputes and generally to help you and your loved ones work through any bumps in the road during hospitalization. Say you have been in the hospital for three days, and you suddenly need to consult the patient relations department, but at the time of admission, you forgot to get their number. It doesn't matter. Just pick up the phone and dial the hospital operator, who will be happy to connect you. Let the patient relations staff know about your observations, especially if they are less than favorable or identify a danger. Is there mold growing in your shower? Are the floors wet in the bathroom or hallway? Is equipment left out where it constitutes a tripping hazard? Are noise levels preventing you from resting? If you pre-register, be sure to obtain the contact information and bring the needed phone extension with you to the hospital. It is worth your while to take care of these small details and have them under your belt before you begin recovering from a painful procedure or are under the influence of pain medications. Be sure to give the patient relations phone number to your advocate, the person who will need to intervene on your behalf in case of an emergency.

Patient relations specialists are usually not available after hours, so a problem that arises in the evening or over a weekend may need to be addressed by a "house officer" or other after-hours representative of the administration. Inquire ahead of time about the after-hours policy and find out whom to contact in an urgent situation. In serious situations, there are *always* resources available to the patient or her representative even after regular business hours. Fortunately, all discussions with patient relations personnel are confidential unless you request otherwise.

Hospital Administration

The administrator of a hospital is responsible for the development, strategic planning, and personnel management for that institution. His department helps the hospital run efficiently and seeks to attain peak performance from all staff members. Even though the public is largely unaware of this potential ally, the hospital administrator is a powerful resource for patients because he can make instant decisions, alter hospital policy to accommodate a patient's needs, and effect immediate change. While it is often most effective to handle questions or problems by consulting those closest to the situation (nurses, physicians, patient relations and social services), some circumstances or emergency situations—such as removing a MD from a case, dealing with an impaired staff member, or handling the deteriorating condition of a patient—may arise that requires decisions from a higher authority.

Remember the story of Lewis Blackman in Chapter Two—a healthy 15-year-old boy who exhibited glaringly obvious signs of shock, which were under-assessed by medical residents? Even the patient's mother's frantic reaction to her son's sudden decline did not alert them to the serious nature of his condition. This type of incident (especially one that involves a younger otherwise healthy patient) is the kind that warrants a quick move up the chain of command. In the competitive environment of healthcare delivery, successful patient outcomes are the paramount goal for administrators; they *need* our continued business to ensure their institution's financial stability. Good customer service has finally moved higher up on every hospital's priority list.

Administrators have a huge responsibility to guarantee that there is a process for evaluating the quality of care they provide. In short, they represent the bottom line for quality control assurance. The public needs to let administrators know that they do not expect them to hide behind boardroom doors, but to be accessible when they haven't yet received a satisfactory response from others. Patients have the right to expect these administrators to personally address safety issues and to act as powerful advocates for quality medical care by stepping in when serious situations arise. The benefit here is two-fold: the patient goes home in good condition, and the hospital is given the opportunity to evaluate how its performance can be improved. A recent study by Thomas *et al* suggests that having hospital executives attend rounds may have a positive impact on the "safety culture" in hospitals. In other words, having administrators walking around the hospital interacting with the nursing staff and asking specifically about "near-misses" they may have witnessed, events that resulted in harm to a patient, and the staff's ideas for preventing adverse events improves communication and reinforces to the staff that the hospital places patient safety high on their list of priorities. Don't be shy about asking the nursing staff if the administration includes them in patient protection strategies and let administrators know that you have heard about healthcare executives being included in rounds.

Convey the message that you consider them a valuable component of any hospital's safety plan and that you are more than willing to share your experiences with administrators.

The administrator's office is just a phone call away. These people have both the duty and the authority to respond to your needs. Remember, though, that for true emergencies or serious conflicts, the nursing supervisor or other staff members can contact the House Supervisor or Administration Supervisor. It is their job to assume responsibility for problems or emergencies in the absence of an administrator; they are the extension of the hospital administration during the evening, weekends, and holidays. When they aren't readily available, an on-call administrator can consult with members of the staff 24 hours a day either in person or via phone or email.

Whenever there are problems or dangers of a caliber that represents a "systems failure"—meaning that the current procedures are flawed and the same problems will occur over and over again until the specific conditions that led to the error are modified—you must make administrators aware of them. I can give you a small example of how a systems error occurs by recounting something that happened in my own dental practice. Recently, a patient came in for a filling on tooth #3. The decay was on the occlusal (or biting surface), which would also give it a listing of "O." Consequently, the front desk would schedule this as "Comp #3-O." The new assistant, who was unaware of the nomenclature in my office, interpreted the number incorrectly and set up for us to work on tooth #30 instead. I might have started drilling the wrong tooth, but I caught the mistake right away because it is my routine to confirm the tooth and surface before I begin. Even though no harm was done, I realized that this was my own version of a "systems flaw"- a situation which, if left in place, could allow for the wrong tooth to be operated on. My solution was relatively simple: we would now enter into the computer the occlusal surface of a tooth as OCC, not just O. The procedure for tooth #3 would now read #3-OCC, making it impossible to mistake it for another number.

Obviously, my office represents a small "system" and one that is easily modified. A hospital represents an amazingly complex and convoluted environment where solutions to systems failures are much more difficult. System flaws in the healthcare setting can be far-reaching and are often responsible for such serious events such as handing out the wrong medication, leaving instruments in patients during surgery, performing surgery on the wrong body parts and spreading deadly infection from patient to patient. In order to identify and solve a systems flaw, administrators need to identify the "root causes" of an event by backtracking and retracing every single step that led to the error and then evaluate every possible contributing factor. In a well-publicized case that resulted in the wrong female patient having a heart procedure that was meant for another patient, *seventeen* contributing root causes were identified.

Reporting near misses is also important because even though no one was injured at that time, and even though a patient dodged a bullet (sometimes through pure luck), there is still a flaw in the system that allowed the error to reach the patient. Were you handed the wrong medication, given the wrong dose of a medication, or was the wrong bag hung on your IV pole? Was the mistake somehow caught before the medication or fluid was administered? Did your nurse ever walk into your room with medication in a cup only to look down and realize that it was meant for another patient? One might be tempted to think, "Wow, I have a great nurse who caught the mistake. She is really on the ball." While it may indeed be true that your nurse is top-notch, you must still insist that she fill out a medication incident form so that quality control personnel can evaluate what allowed the wrong medication to reach your bedside in the first place. Even near misses represent serious flaws in the system, and they must be evaluated and dealt with; the next patient might not be so lucky. When you ponder what difference an individual can really have on patient safety, it becomes increasingly clear that patients and their advocates are in the ideal position to be a driving force for healthcare quality.

Department Heads/Service Heads

The departments or "services" of Pediatrics, Surgery, Orthopedics and others all have physicians (called department heads or heads of service) who work in a supervisory role and assume responsibility for overseeing the doctors working in their department. If you have a disagreement or a dispute with your physician or with his treatment plan, if communication between you and your doctor is poor or non-existent, or if any other situation arises that makes you feel that you must go over your doctor's head, you can contact the department head for advice.

Looking back, my husband and I wish we had consulted the head of the Orthopedics Department during our crisis. Our daughter had been admitted to the ICU with a life-threatening condition. My husband and I were convinced it was an infection related to a bone biopsy that had been performed several days earlier. The orthopedic surgeon who was called in to consult took a perfunctory look at the incision site and declared that he was sure this was not an infection. The more we insisted on other tests to rule out the possibility of infection, the deeper he dug in his heels. In my opinion, his own ego, and not our daughter's health, was his primary motivation for refusing to budge. Days later, with our daughter literally dying from toxic shock syndrome, we had to threaten to contact an attorney and bring a lawsuit before he would agree to do a minor surgical exploration of the biopsy site. This procedure confirmed what we had suspected all along—the biopsy site was badly infected and the resulting osteomyelitis, or deep bone infection, had led to dangerous bacteria being introduced into Kate's bloodstream. We will always wonder if a new perspective from a doctor with authority over this particular surgeon would have offered us a more timely and accurate diagnosis.

My husband and I will never know if consulting with the head of the Orthopedic Department would have helped Kate, but we don't want others to miss the opportunity to contact a resource that could save their life and alleviate their suffering. The Patient Relations department can assist you in locating the correct department head. Contact the individual by phone or in person and ask that she examine the patient and review the treatment plan as soon as possible. She should also be able to make recommendations for obtaining a second opinion or changing you to a new physician in the department. If your physician is the department head, you need to contact the hospital administrator to help facilitate your request for another opinion.

Social Services

Social Services personnel function as coordinators between the patient, the healthcare team, and a multitude of community resources that may be available to patients. Patients and their families will want to stay in close communication with its staff members to find out about necessary services and referrals. Social Services staff members are available to aid people before, during, and after a hospital visit. A decline in health can cause intense feelings of anxiety, despair, and fear, and Social Services is there to help people cope with the emotional, physical, and financial problems often associated with illness and hospitalization.

Responsibilities of the Social Services department may include locating financial assistance programs, arranging for individual or group counseling, and assisting in nursing home or assisted living arrangements. Social Services personnel are often able to aid in securing transportation for patients, in providing home healthcare referrals, and in securing durable medical equipment. Social workers help link patients to resources that are made available to them by their communities, such as meal delivery programs, hospice care, support groups, and programs or agencies to aid people who are unable to afford medical expenses not covered by insurance. For example, if you need a hearing aid or an expensive pair of glasses, you can be directed to community groups or charities that may have funds earmarked for such necessities. Social workers can often initiate contact with appropriate agencies, start the process for you, and they will communicate any requirements, paperwork or fees that need to be addressed.

A hospital stay can go on much longer than expected, which often leads to depression and confusion, especially in elderly patients. Unexpectedly, a parent, aunt or uncle might need to be transferred to a nursing home or a rehabilitation facility; the family will naturally be in a quandary about finding the best site. A patient's health may deteriorate to the point that he is no longer able to care for himself. Home care is needed, but the family has no idea how to find a loving caregiver. Social workers hear these problems every day. To be of help, they strive to remain focused on the overall picture so they can both address the many-faceted needs of patients and provide comfort and hope in the midst of tragedy and pain.

On a more interactive level, patients can turn to Social Services personnel to help open the lines of communication between themselves and their caregivers, to help them express questions and concerns, and to facilitate between patients (or their representatives) and physicians during family meetings. Social workers have access to medical records, so they can help translate confusing medical lingo into terms patients can understand and then show them how to voice their grievances appropriately. Social workers are tireless problem solvers whose main goal is to help patients and their families cope with feelings of helplessness and isolation during their hospital stay, especially if a patient has to listen to a bitterly disappointing diagnosis, if he is told he has been a victim of a medical error, or if there is a decline in status that necessitates immediate family decisions.

Medical Center Director/Chief Operating Officer or COO

Most institutions employ a director or Chief Operating Officer (COO), who works closely with administrators to direct operational issues facing the hospital. The COO is the level directly over the head of the administration, and if you are not satisfied after an encounter with an administrator, this is the person to contact next. The COO is the medical counterpart to the CEO of a Fortune 500 company. The director or COO implements policy, ensures strong communication and cooperation between administration and medical staff, works with city and state officials to help meet the health needs of the community, secures new sources of revenue for the medical center and helps the institution with quality control issues by being attuned to the complaints or dissatisfaction of both staff members and patients.

In general, any time you want to contact the hospital administration, send a letter detailing your experience to the COO. This is akin to calling the head of a car company if you have a serious problem with your vehicle. Most likely, a consumer would start by communicating his dissatisfaction to the salesman. If there was no progress, he could work his way up the chain of command by speaking with the dealership management and then the regional manager. If none of this works and he is still stuck with a lemon, he can go straight to the top and let the national office know that he still has five years to pay on a car that won't start on cold mornings. Maybe they will shrug off your letter or call. But if they receive enough complaints, they cannot fail to see that there is a real problem. I know several people who have had manufacturers buy their car back from them because the problems they experienced were serious and ongoing. Car manufacturers know that customer satisfaction is vital to their growth and profits. Now it's time to remind healthcare administrators that the trust and support of the public is vital to their wellbeing, too.

If you cannot find a resolution to a valid complaint, if you feel that the administration is looking the other way about a problem you know is serious, and especially if you feel that other patients are at risk of finding themselves in the same plight as you, then it is especially important to contact the COO. On the flip side, positive experiences such as a superior caregiver, staff members who went out of their way to assist you, and special features of the hospital that increased your comfort level are also worth communicating to the top administrators. The patient relations department can provide you with the name of the director and the mailing address to send correspondence since it is unlikely that the COO will be willing to interact directly at the bedside with patients or family members –although you can always ask.

It is probably most efficient to contact the COO in writing.

Clearly state the nature of your problem. Include your name, date of hospitalization, medical record number, physician's name, and the unit you were in. It is especially important to include any issues that impacted your hospital stay and any ideas or suggestions that would have improved it. One situation involving my own mother warranted a letter to the COO. The nurses were so short staffed during my mother's stay for dehydration that they stopped keeping track of her urine and bowel output. When I realized what was going on, I asked how they could possibly be adjusting her IV fluids correctly to make up for her loss of fluid if they weren't recording her intake and output. One nurse's solution was to hand my mother a piece of paper and a pen and have her measure her own fluid intake and urine output and write it down on a piece of paper left in the bathroom. I felt that the COO needed to be informed about both the staffing issue and the "self-serve" approach that this nurse recommended, which was highly unprofessional and certainly chock-full of opportunity for errors. I doubt that this was an approved customer satisfaction strategy. In your own letter, state that you are requesting a written response. Keep a copy of your communication, and if you don't receive a timely reply, follow up with a phone call. Even if you do not deal with the COO directly, having the top administrator apprised of the situation will help keep everyone on his or her toes.

The COO or director of a hospital is another powerful healthcare decision-maker. Whenever anything truly serious or life-threatening occurs during your hospitalization, it is important to communicate it to the top administrator because he can implement meaningful changes as a result of your information. Taking the time to contact this individual directly will alert him to areas that need evaluation and improvement. It is a lot harder to brush complaints aside as isolated incidents when a number of patients all seem to be voicing the same concerns. And remember, incidents that happen over and over could very well be an indication of systems flaws that will only be resolved by a change in hospital procedure mandated by a top administrator.

Proactive patients and their representatives will be fro
lysts for healthcare reform simply by taking the time an
notify the people at the top about the quality of the care the
whether positive or negative. A disappointing hospital experience is
not just your personal problem, and your only recourse does not have
to be complaining to your next-door neighbor or co-workers when
you get home. By communicating and complaining effectively to
those who can do something about it, you will help everyone. This
goes way beyond just thinking of yourself. It is an opportunity for
you to make a meaningful contribution to the greater good by taking
action to improve the quality of healthcare for all.

Infection Control Specialist

The Infection Control Specialist manages the hospital's infection
control program and implements the policies that minimize the risk
of nosocomial (hospital-acquired) infections for patients, visitors
and staff members. You can expect infection control personnel to be
involved whenever there is an outbreak of infection (i.e., two or more
patients with the same infective organism) so they can check for deficiencies in infection control policies or procedures, when a patient is
critically ill from an infection acquired either inside or outside of the
hospital, if a patient death leaves any unanswered questions about
whether not infection was a contributing factor, or if organisms
appearing in the hospital are resistant to the antibiotics normally able
to combat them.

Infections are an absolute scourge in hospitals. They quickly
emerge as a threat to every patient, and they need to be identified and
contained as quickly as possible. Your nurse and doctor are on the
front line; they will diagnose and treat any infection you may acquire.
But the infection control specialist will work tirelessly to look for
the root cause of your infection and be sure that other patients are
protected.

Infection control professionals make use of several means to reduce the incidence of infection:

1. They must first educate themselves and others in the institution about the infectious process so everyone has a conceptual understanding of the mechanisms that cause infection.

2. They perform surveillance (observation and identification) to study the possible ways that infections travel and how well staff members are following established control policies.

3. They use the raw data from infection statistics so they can distribute the collected information to hospital staff members, educating them about the prevention and containment of infection.

4. They modify or alter the infection control policies if they are found to be deficient.

5. They are available to speak to patients or their families to explain the infectious process and to suggest ways that patients can protected themselves.

Given these duties, you would want to contact them if you develop an infection; observe poor infection control measures in your caregivers (which you will be more than able to assess after reading Chapter Three); want a professional assessment of the status of your immune system or your risk of infection from roommates, visitors, or staff; or if you develop an infection that appears soon after you return home so they will know that it could have been initiated in their facility (again, see Chapter Three).

Once Infection Control Specialists identify an outbreak of infection, they begin an investigation. Even if you acquire an infection that appears to be an isolated occurrence, you can still request that the infection control specialist investigate the possible sources and report any findings to you. Infection control staff are busy people, so be sure you don't get lost in the shuffle. If you don't hear back in a timely manner, call them again. They are invaluable to patients because they can immediately implement new safety measures to protect you, evaluate the system in place for flaws or deficiencies and correct them immediately, interview staff members about their infection control techniques and train the staff to prevent future outbreaks. An example of the ability of Infection Control professionals to save lives was demonstrated at Johns Hopkins Hospital in 2004. The medical intensive care unit at Hopkins had one of the highest rates of catheter-related bloodstream infections in the entire hospital. Six years of studying the problem and the institution of several new evidence-based protocols resulted in a 75 percent reduction in bloodstream infection rates. A major contributor to this success story was determined infection control officers who were willing to spend years collecting data, looking at statistics from other hospitals, and performing close surveillance after new strategies were implemented to make sure they really worked. Recently, Johns Hopkins took its patient safety efforts to another level by sharing its impressive improvement data with other ICU's across the country. As a result, central line bloodstream infections in many of the other ICU's *dropped to zero.* Further proof that such results are not pie-in-the-sky dreams; they represent realistic goals.

The Center for Disease Control reports that two million patients will develop a hospital-acquired infection each year and 90,000 people will die as a result. Ninety-thousand! The numbers are staggering, and I feel strongly that all patients who develop an infection in the hospital should request a meeting with the infection control specialist employed by their facility. It may seem like an annoying way to consume your time, but it is important. When you are ill, it's easy to be self-absorbed. "All I want to do is get better and get out of here. Let the next guy worry about himself." We must, however, develop an altruistic mindset and to get in touch with the right people when we observe an endemic problem. As a patient, you have a unique perspective, and you may even have vital information or observations that other staff members can't impart or won't share due to their fear of seeming critical of a coworker.

Looking at the above statistics, it is obvious that we need these specially trained staff members to step in and monitor each and every situation that involves infection if we are to have any real chance of reducing these staggering numbers. Your nurse or the Patient Relations department can help you make the right calls. Remember to ask pointedly if your infection meets the criteria to be classified as a nosocomial infection (see Chapter Three) and request that an investigation be conducted to identify its possible sources.

Every patient has the right to be cared for by staff members who are practicing adequate infection control measures, and it is the responsibility of the infection control specialist to evaluate and monitor their activities. All hospitals in the United States are required to have written infection control programs in place and well-defined procedures by which they regularly evaluate the success of their efforts. The ability to quickly identify and classify nosocomial infections correctly is a vital component of any patient safety program. If you develop a nosocomial infection, ask that it be included in the hospital's infection statistics. Patients can also report infections directly to their state hospital licensing boards or to the Joint Commission.

Hospital Licensing and Certification

This is one of the first government agencies that patients can approach to report errors and deficiencies and the first group not employed directly by the hospital. The purpose of licensing and certification agencies is to improve the quality of care in our communities by ensuring that state health and safety laws are being implemented. These laws establish the criteria that hospitals must meet to keep their licenses, and each state employs investigators who make sure that minimum performance standards are met. They visit medical facilities either on a regular basis or when a specific problem is reported to them. Licensing and certification agencies are administered under the auspices of State Health Services departments (often called Department of Health Services), which, of course, can make them subject to political and budget restrictions. Individual states legislate

their own health and safety laws for the public's protection in
by visiting and inspecting medical facilities during the construction,
maintenance and operation of hospitals and surgery centers. By definition, then, it is the licensing and certification agencies that are in
charge of the front line oversight of healthcare institutions.

State hospital licensing boards are equipped to investigate consumer complaints, but most people have no idea that this resource
is available to them. While this is not their main focus, they are
equipped to deal directly with the public and to address concerns.
Ideally, they would be contacted by the hospitals themselves each and
every time a serious, unanticipated event results in patient injury or
death. If the hospital is not willing to step up to the plate and report
an issue, then open the phone book, look under government agencies, and make the call yourself. Whenever the hospital isn't doing
an adequate investigation or not sharing the information it has with
you, the licensing board can assist you in getting the ball rolling and
obtaining information.

With certain occurrences, the licensing agencies expect hospitals to report them voluntarily. For example, a district administrator from the California Department of Health Services informed me
that outbreaks of disease and unusual circumstances such as unex-
plained deaths or fires should be immediately reported by the institution. When I asked her if she felt that hospitals were reporting all the
events that they should, it was clear from her response that she did
not. Why? Because it made them look bad, and in our era of hospital
"report cards" being published in local newspapers, who wants to be
the only hospital in town coming clean with its faults? The supervisor told me, "We can only investigate what we know about, and the
reporting is essentially voluntary." Most of the complaints landing
on her desk originate from hospital employees or from patients themselves, not from hospital administration, which tells you how important it is for the public to speak up.

To make a complaint, contact the Department of Health Services or the state capitol to be directed to the division that inspects

hospitals. In California, for example, patients should contact the Licensing and Certification Division, which will direct them to the appropriate district office. Right at the beginning, ask for guidance and follow their directions exactly, keeping a copy for your records; this is a bureaucratic agency so complaints can be misplaced or filed incorrectly. Once a complaint is properly registered, the investigator will speak to the patient or his or her representative and then to staff members at the medical facility. Under these circumstances, the hospital cannot refuse to participate in the investigation, and the investigator will review the patient's medical record. Complaints are deemed "substantiated" or "unsubstantiated" with unsubstantiated cases being closed with no further investigation and no opportunity for appeal.

Investigators have the authority to issue "deficiencies," which are admonitions about care that does not meet a minimum standard; they are based on specific guidelines in each state's health and safety laws. One of the main reasons to contact a licensing board is that it does have some power to make hospitals change the way they do business. If nothing else, it keeps statistics on the numbers and types of complaints it receives. After receiving a deficiency, an institution is required to submit a plan of correction to be implemented within a specified amount of time. When an investigation is complete, the licensing agency prepares a report. A report or summary of the agency's findings are not routinely shared with the complainant; the individual making the complaint is usually only notified of the specific code violation if a deficiency is found. The Code of Regulations in your state may grant access to these reports as a provision of law, so check.

We desperately wanted to see the report to read what our daughter's doctors would say when they were questioned in person by an outside agency with authority over them instead of by two tired, disillusioned parents. What were their thought processes when they were making decisions and determining a course of treatment that had gone wrong? Whatever investigation the hospital was conducting, they weren't telling us anything, and this seemed the only way to piece together the disjointed string of events that had led to such a disastrous result. We were the ones who had suffered and had to live with the consequences, yet we were being left out of the picture. After months went by, we finally received a copy of our complaint report with the names of the doctors blacked out, but it was still incredibly valuable to us to see in black and white the rationale behind the decisions that resulted in a flawed treatment plan. The most disturbing aspect of the document was that only one doctor was willing to go on record stating that he disagreed with the initial assessment and tried to get further testing ordered. Every other physician who had expressed any doubts during the days that we were desperately trying to find the cause of Kate's illness suddenly developed amnesia, circled the wagons, and, albeit reluctantly, defended the orthopedic surgeon.

I believe that it is important to try to insist on seeing the report. State laws or freedom of information acts may be your best ally in this, so do your homework and be prepared to quote any specific laws or statutes that may allow you access. My husband and I never received the resolution we sought from the Licensing and Certification agency, which was that the doctors and the hospital would be sanctioned. However, contacting the Department of Health Services was important anyway. We wanted an impartial third party to review our situation, officially document our complaint, interview Kate's physicians, and finally have them explain their actions "for the record."

State licensing boards have limited power and authority. Don't expect a team of investigators to come storming into the hospital threatening to shut it down because you have given them a list of complaints. Be prepared for the fact that the doctor who missed an obvious diagnosis and thereby caused extreme physical and emotional harm to your family will probably not be held accountable in any way. Even though licensing investigators don't work for the hospital, their bosses may be pressured to protect hospitals for political reasons; people in high places or those running for office may have an interest in the healthcare system appearing better and safer than it really is. This has long been a criticism of these agencies—the fact that they are not truly independent.

An important lesson I learned dealing with Licensing and Certification is that patients and their advocates must learn to recognize the need for documenting their case. The first thing the investigator asked me was if we had any photos or video of Kate's leg when it had been swollen and red many days earlier. I would never have thought of pictures or video on my own, but it does bring up a good point. Pictures or video of a wound, for instance, can show a process of worsening signs and symptoms. Since state investigators are often notified after a serious event, they may miss the opportunity to ask families to document their situation. Patients and their advocates who disagree with their treatment or lack thereof need to document any relevant clinical manifestations. In such cases, a single picture or video could be worth more than a thousand words.

Bringing these issues out from behind closed doors is what will ultimately lead to timely solutions. While an individual complaint to a licensing board may not lead to immediate change, there is power in numbers, and a single piece of information can ultimately have great impact when it is evaluated with other similar information. Your complaint could end up being the one that causes an institution to initiate important changes that can save thousand of others.

Medical Boards

The Federation of State Medical Boards consists of 68 member boards whose primary goal is to protect the public by regulating physicians and other allied healing professionals such as physical therapists, podiatrists, opticians, and so on. The general duties of each state medical board are to oversee the licensing of physicians, regulate the practice of medicine and discipline those who violate the Medical Practice Act. Each state has its own legal statutes that govern the provisions of this act. Why is this important to you? Because, theoretically, it affords you protection from injury, ensures increased healthcare quality, and establishes a baseline for evaluating established treatment standards.

Patients, family members, and hospital personnel may all file a complaint with their State Medical Board (often there is an 800 number). Information about the mailing addresses and requirements in every state can be obtained via the Internet or by phoning the state capital and asking for the State Medical Board. Once a complaint is made, a preliminary assessment is done, and if the case has merit, it is referred for further investigation. As long as there is no flagrant violation (such as sexual abuse by a doctor), the investigator can use his own subjective judgment about whether to proceed with an inquiry. Once the investigation is complete (the process can be long and tedious - ours took over six months), several outcomes are possible. A case can be closed without action, there can be administrative sanctions such as suspension of a license, or the case can be referred to the Attorney General or the local District Attorney for legal action.

Medical boards often provide information to consumers regarding the number of license suspensions and revocations and about large malpractice judgments in their state. Smaller settlements (under $30,000), which are generally considered nuisance suits, and arbitration awards, are not disclosed to the public. The National Practitioner Data Bank, which tracks the disciplinary history of physicians, is, unfortunately, still inaccessible to the public, and there is even talk of abolishing it altogether.

Public advocacy groups have long criticized medical boards for their inefficiency and their potential for physician-to-physician bias when investigating complaints. According to critics, their first loyalty is to the doctors and preserving the medical profession's image, not to protecting patients. In 1993, the California Department of Justice responded to years of complaints and a *60 Minutes* expose about the California Medical Board and wanted to conduct an investigation, but they couldn't convince the Attorney General's office to do it because of a potential conflict of interest; certain staff members employed by their office were currently investigating cases referred by the Medical Board. The California Highway Patrol was asked to step in as the investigative agency next in line to conduct an unbiased investigation. In a scathing report, the CHP exposed a number of serious problems with the Board's policies and administration. In recognition of the criticism, the Board attempted to head off trouble by voting for reforms including granting access to information by medical consumers, additional sanctions for physicians, and an improved medical quality review system.

California has a greater number of licensed and practicing physicians than any other state. Using statistics from 2003-2005, California ranks twenty-third in the nation in serious disciplinary actions with approximately 363 prejudicial actions per year for 105,766 practicing physicians. California has imposed a very high burden of proof for cases before the Medical Board, and our letter from them closing out our complaint stated that the standards in California for violation of the Medical Practice Act required "clear and convincing evidence. This is a higher standard of proof than that of most civil proceedings, including malpractice suits." A brochure available on the Medical Board of California Web site states: . . . "If the Board finds that the treatment fell below the standard of care but does not represent gross negligence, the complaint will be closed but will be maintained on file for the Board's future reference." Think about it. In California, it is harder to prove a violation to the State Medical Board than to prevail in a court of law as part of a malpractice suit and unless your complaint involves "gross negligence" it will be shelved. It's no wonder that so few complaints ever lead to action by medical boards. Nevertheless, it is still important to lodge a complaint. Even if a complaint does not result in the disciplinary action you expect, the numbers and the data are being collected and evaluated, and they are increasingly available to the public and to the legislature. With approximately 40 percent of Americans reporting that they, or someone they know, have been injured by our healthcare system, it is obvious that there is a troubling disparity between the number of injuries and the number of doctors disciplined.

Medical Board investigations represent predominantly a peer-review system. This means that physicians assess the judgments and actions of their fellow physicians, creating the potential for bias. Many feel that the long-standing policy of "self-policing" by physicians and the honor system of reporting information to State Medical Boards and other agencies literally brings chances of improving health care in this country to a standstill. But when warranted, it is vital to spend the time wading through this process because without statistics on the true numbers of patient injuries, it becomes virtually impossible to accurately assess the scope of the problem, to make a case to hospitals or legislators for increased patient safety resources, or to find meaningful solutions.

The Joint Commission (Formerly the Joint Commission on Accreditation of Health Care Organizations)

"Do you have a complaint about the quality of care at a
Joint Commission-accredited health care organization?
The Joint Commission wants to know about it."
—*Joint Commission Website, 2007*

The Joint Commission is a private, non-profit group that functions as the nation's leading healthcare accrediting body and acts as a "quasi-regulatory organization." The mission of the Commission is to improve the quality of care by accredited hospitals and make recommendations for improvement that set the standards for care. Literally, the Joint Commission knocks on the hospital door, and then conducts a complete evaluation of all the systems and issues a report on how they are doing compared with other institutions. Since we have no comprehensive federal agency that can mandate immediate safety measures, the Commission is considered the main driving force behind official patient safety efforts. However, participation in the review process by healthcare organizations is voluntary, it is funded almost entirely by the institutions being evaluated, and some of its board members are hospital executives. Naturally, this leads people to question its ability to be completely unbiased.

Medicare and other third-party payers have recently forced the hand of healthcare institutions by making accreditation by this organization a requirement in order to be able to be reimbursed for services rendered. Even though the Joint Commission is an approved accreditation agency, it still has limited ability to impose any real sanctions on the hospitals it evaluates. Until recently, hospitals knew well in advance when they would receive an official visit from evaluators, which is akin to cleaning your house when you know *Good Housekeeping Magazine* is coming by for a photo shoot. Human nature being what it is, very few of us can sustain the same degree of effort when we know no one will be checking. In response to this criticism, Joint Commission shifted to unannounced surveys in 2006. According to President Dr. Dennis O'Leary, "The new accreditation process creates the expectation that each accredited organization be in compliance with 100 percent of the Joint Commission's standards 100 percent of the time."

The Joint Commission evaluates more than 19,500 healthcare organizations in the United States, including hospitals, managed care networks, healthcare organizations that provide home care, long-term care facilities, behavioral health care, laboratory services, and ambulatory care centers. The Joint Commission offers both information and services to increase public awareness about the quality of care they receive. It accepts complaints from the public regarding such issues as medication errors, patient suicides, restraint deaths, wrong-site surgery, transfusion errors, falls and delays in treatment. (See their Web site for a complete listing.) Issues within the scope of the Joint Commission (www.jointcommission.org) standards include patient rights, patient care, safety, infection control, medication use, errors, and security.

The Joint Commission will not investigate complaints against unaccredited organizations. If you have a problem with an accredited organization however, contact them by fax 630-792-5636, by e-mail (complaint@jointcommission.org), by using a toll free number 800-994-6610, or by a Quality Incident Report form that you can print out from their Web site. You may also mail the above mentioned form, or a letter stating the name and address of the institution, the nature of your complaint, and whether you request confidentiality. However, an investigator I spoke to said that requesting complete confidentiality might limit the scope of the investigation.

When healthcare organizations undergo a "full survey," there used to be an opportunity for family, patients, advocates, and advocacy groups to participate in a Public Information Interview, because the dates of the visits were announced in advance. Now, with unannounced surveys, it is much more difficult for the public to participate in the process, although the Joint Commission does check during its survey how hospitals inform the public of their right to make a complaint to the Commission. As it stands now, the patient or family member would have to hear that there are surveyors on-site and call the hospital administration to schedule an interview with representatives from the Joint Commission. This puts the entire burden on the individual to be in ongoing contact with the hospital to determine if a survey is occurring. Contacting the Joint Commission will tell you the date of the last survey, which can give you an idea if a new survey is on the horizon.

Once a complaint is received, Joint Commission's investigation begins with a review of any past complaints and the current Accreditation Survey Report on file. It can take one or more actions in response to each complaint:

1. For serious concerns such as an incident that resulted in an unexpected patient death, the Joint Commission can conduct an unannounced, on-site evaluation of the organization.

2. It can ask the organization to provide a written response to the complaint.

3. It can include the complaint in its own database of statistics to help track the performance of the healthcare organization over time.

4. It may review the complaint at the next scheduled accreditation survey if it is scheduled in the near future.

5. In extreme circumstances, it can downgrade accreditation status to "conditional accreditation" or "preliminary denial of accreditation" if serious deficiencies are found.

The Joint Commission also has a Sentinel Event Policy to encourage institutions to self-report specific adverse events and to conduct root cause analyses to reduce the risk of future sentinel event occurrences. A sentinel event is one that has resulted in an unanticipated death, a major permanent loss of function not related to the patient's original illness, a patient suicide in a setting where the patient was supposed to receive around-the-clock care and therefore observation, infant abduction or release to the wrong family, rape, blood transfusions involving major blood group incompatibilities, or surgery on the wrong patient or the wrong body part. The root cause analysis is the process of backtracking and determining what contributed to the disastrous results. Interestingly, the Joint Commission has listed communication glitches as the number one contributing factor in sentinel events. Other root causes include faulty orientation and training, incomplete patient assessment, staffing issues, lack of compliance with established procedures, and interruption in the continuity of care. (See the Web site for a complete listing.)

The Joint Commission becomes aware of sentinel events when they are self-reported by hospitals (65.7 percent), by the media (7.6 percent), through complaints (12.5 percent), during accreditation surveys (8.5 percent) and from agencies such as Medicare and Medicaid (5.8 percent). While it is admirable that the Joint Commission has established such a tracking system, patients need to be aware that since it started keeping track in 1995, the Commission has only 4,234 sentinel events listed in its database, even though we know that there have been hundreds of thousands of reportable situations. Since we know that 30,000 people will die each year from preventable medication errors and 90,000 will die from hospital-acquired infections, one can only conclude that the number of sentinel events being tracked is shockingly low. But that could all change tomorrow if patients knew how important it was to share their stories. I would hope, after the release of this book that the number of sentinel events reported to the Joint Commission takes a huge leap forward. This organization *wants* to know about your experiences; all you have to do is to want to tell them and realize how simple it is to do it. Once patients know they can add their experiences to the pool of information, we won't have to rely on such small amounts of data to help find solutions to the serious problem of medical errors.

The Joint Commission does release some information about complaints received by accredited organizations. Their performance reports on individual facilities can be obtained free-of-charge by calling or writing to the commission or through their Web site (look under Quality Check on the Web site). After they complete their review of a complaint, they will inform the complainant of any actions they have taken as a result of the complaint, but they do not make their findings available. So, their final actions are made public, but the details of the investigation and any relevant discoveries are withheld. For this very reason, many patients find the Joint Commission experience frustrating, even infuriating.

The Joint Commission is far from a perfect solution and has been criticized for being too lenient in their evaluations and for not taking more disciplinary actions against healthcare facilities when they don't meet the standard of care. A preferred solution might be a completely independent, government-funded accrediting organization with greater resources and more power to effect immediate and mandatory nationwide change, such as the recently implemented Joint Commission policy of marking of surgical sites ahead of time or outlawing unlabeled medications that look alike to sit in cups in the operating room just waiting for someone to mix them up. As it stands though, the Joint Commission represents one of the few nationwide systems in place to track complaints and sentinel events.

Will reporting incidents to the Joint Commission provide patients, family members, or hospital personnel with the much-needed sense of vindication and accountability they desire? Probably not. But without individual incidents being systematically logged into a central database, we will never be able to ascertain the true magnitude of the problems and dangers. Without the raw data to evaluate the true scope of medical error, the solutions we search for will remain elusive. Again we come back to the altruistic motive—you may not be the one who is helped this time around, but a safer healthcare system will certainly benefit you or a loved one at a future date. A 2002 news release from the Joint Commission spoke of the roles each and every group involved in our medical system must assume if we are to achieve our goal of safe and effective healthcare. The last line of the press release stated the necessary role of patients and their advocates very clearly. According to the Joint Commission, individual patients and their advocates have the responsibility of "monitoring and participating in their care."

Media

The power of the written word is clearly evident when you look at the statistics from the Joint Commission listing the sources for sentinel event identification. Each year, a certain number of sentinel events come to the attention of the Joint Commission from media coverage; it is evident how valuable a resource the media can be. Contacting them is usually a last resort and is often turned to when all other attempts at dealing with a hospital over a serious problem has failed.

In my case, it was an investigator from the Joint Commission who first suggested to me that involving the media is a powerful means to an end. She advised me to find out the names of writers who cover medical stories for our local paper. Often, they will report a variety of issues, but they may have a special interest in specific subjects. I have contacted several responsive and receptive reporters after reading pieces they wrote in which certain stories were similar to ours.

The information you provide may result in important media coverage to help alert the public to ways they can keep themselves safe. And since media stories that appear in smaller publications could be picked up by larger ones, you don't have to start with the *New York Times*. Begin with a local paper and work your way up.

There is a flip side to this. Some people feel uncomfortable appearing or being quoted in the news. In addition, they frequently find that parts of the story, which they thought were crucial, were edited out of the piece completely. They have virtually no control over the tone, length or style of the media story once they report it.

I have read and collected literally thousands of media stories over the years in preparation for this book. Instead of having to search hard for stories to use, which is what I would have expected before writing this book, I usually had at my disposal dozens of tales to fit any situation. I had to sift through them to decide which one best illustrated my point. There is no doubt that our current information age has been a great asset in bringing all kinds of social problems to the public's attention, and healthcare safety has certainly benefited from this phenomenon. The phenomenon of individual patients describing their experiences on Web sites is something that was unthinkable in the near past. Media exposure first bolsters awareness, then focuses public scrutiny on specific issues, and then hopefully leads to a public outcry demanding change.

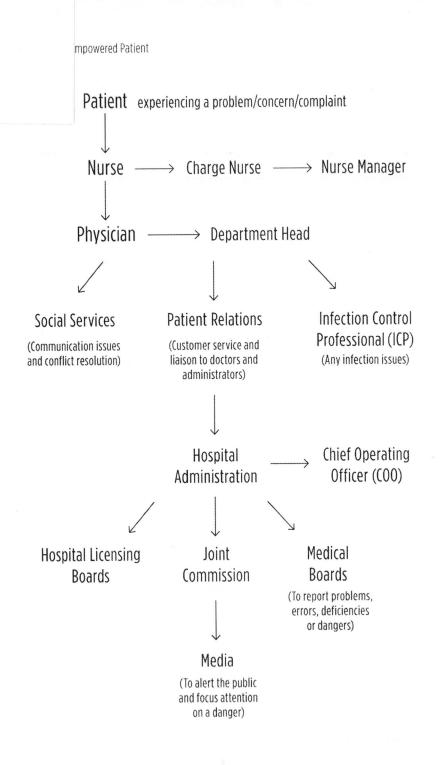

Patient experiencing a problem/concern/complaint

Nurse ⟶ Charge Nurse ⟶ Nurse Manager

Physician ⟶ Department Head

Social Services

(Communication issues
and conflict resolution)

Patient Relations

(Customer service and
liaison to doctors and
administrators)

Infection Control
Professional (ICP)

(Any infection issues)

Hospital
Administration ⟶ Chief Operating
Officer (COO)

Hospital Licensing
Boards

Joint
Commission

Medical
Boards

(To report problems,
errors, deficiencies
or dangers)

Media

(To alert the public
and focus attention
on a danger)

Chapter Seven

Medical Records
The Playbook of Your Life

Even with the recent debate on computerizing medical records, which would allow nationwide access, few of us give much thought to the written records that chronicle our healthcare experiences. Routinely, we take these documents for granted even though they are the point of convergence for every single piece of data relating to our health. An apt metaphor would be, of all things, trucks. Every single man-made item you see or use in a day was transported by truck. The trucking industry touches every aspect of commerce. Medical records are just as central and crucial to health care.

Many people naturally assume that their medical record is inaccessible to them. If they do believe they can get hold of it, they seriously doubt that they can comprehend the vast quantity of technical information it contains. Nevertheless, all patients or their advocates should peruse their medical records; doing so may give them a completely new perspective on their treatment, which may surprise and even shock them.

Federal laws allow virtually all patients to have access to their medical information. The one exception refers to patients with psychiatric illnesses. The physician may feel that certain information could impair the person's mental health. There are, however, few other valid reasons for denying access to medical records. In almost every instance, they should be yours for the asking, although patients assume financial responsibility for the expense of copying their medical records and duplication fees for x-rays and scans.

Having said that, there are a few critical points you should know up front. To illustrate their importance, I will relate how they applied to my life during our medical crisis with our daughter.

YOUR MEDICAL RECORDS MIGHT NOT BE AVAILABLE WHEN YOU NEED THEM

Our first experience requesting medical records came during an unforeseen emergency. Our daughter Kate had just been diagnosed with her first recurrence of malignant eye tumors. As we hastily made plans to travel to a hospital 600 miles away, the ophthalmologist asked us to send copies of Kate's most recent MRI scans to him by overnight mail so he could begin coordinating the complex treatment plan. We were fortunate enough to live five minutes away from the San Francisco hospital where the scans were located.

I immediately phoned the medical center and asked them to have the scans available for me to pick up later in the day. As I entered the Radiation Oncology department, I expected to sign a release and to leave quickly with the scans, but when I arrived, I was told that they were unavailable because they had already been "checked out" by a medical student. Granted, this was 1989, when hard copies were filed in the medical records department and not stored in databases for extended periods of time, so the only way for a student to review cases was to check out a physical file. Of course, I assumed that this person was in some way connected to our daughter's case, but when I asked for the name, it was unfamiliar to us. (Later we were told that the individual was a student who had never actually met us or examined our daughter.) I vaulted between feelings of numbing fear and absolute panic as I explained the desperate situation that made obtaining the scans a priority. I was assured that they would find them ASAP and assume responsibility for sending them overnight mail. Even so, we never stopped worrying that they wouldn't arrive in time to be of value to the new doctor or that they might be lost indefinitely in a bureaucratic snafu.

Fortunately, our computer age now allows for x-rays and scans to be taken digitally and stored in databases or saved on a CD to be given to the patient. This means they should never be "missing" when you need them. Several hospitals in the San Francisco area now store scans in databases for as long as 10 years and will give patients a CD of their scan to be kept at home as an additional backup. X-ray techs I interviewed strongly advised this approach, saying "you never know what could happen" to scans stored in hospital computers – it isn't a completely fail-safe method. At the present time, every hospital I spoke with is providing the CD free of charge. At the time you make the appointment, be sure to ask if your hospital or imaging center is utilizing digital radiography and let them know that you would like a CD. Ask if there will be a fee; perhaps you can bring your own CD and save on costs.

IF SCANS ARE MISSING, FOLLOW UP. YOU SHOULD KNOW WHO IS LOOKING INTO YOUR CASE

After we returned home from the grueling treatments in Los Angeles, I phoned the Medical Records Department to inquire how Kate's scans could possibly have been unavailable to us during a crisis. I was told that all university medical personnel, including students, can view any medical records. In my opinion, "viewing" was not synonymous with "removing." The clerk agreed with my interpretation but explained that the student had probably heard about my daughter's case during rounds or in a lecture and wanted to review the MRI images, but obviously had not followed university rules about viewing scans right there in the department.

FIND OUT WHAT THE OFFICIAL POLICY IS ON THESE MATTERS

The official policy on viewing medical records at this institution is simple. The medical records department has a specially designated area for viewing records. There is a prominent sign stating that they are not to be removed from the premises. A doctor can fill out a request for copies of written records and x-rays to be duplicated, but the official policy states that charts and scans are never to be removed from the medical records department unless specifically needed for the patient's treatment while she is in the hospital. The clerk admitted that the scans "shouldn't have left the premises, but it happens all the time." When I expressed my surprise at the lax enforcement of hospital policy and the ability of just about anyone to view sensitive medical records, I was told "this is a teaching hospital." This convenient, catchall phrase had been tossed at me before in an obvious attempt to put an immediate end to any request for information, explanations, or accountability. Patients are expected to cease all pointed inquiries the moment the phrase "teaching hospital" is handed to them, as if that explained away all breaches of protocol. This time I was not going to be satisfied until I found a way to protect our privacy and assure that Kate's complete medical record was always available.

INQUIRE ABOUT YOUR RIGHTS

I pointedly inquired about my rights in regards to privacy, and when I was initially told that I had little say in the matter, I asked to speak to a supervisor. If you are given information that doesn't make sense or doesn't sound right to you, be sure to write down the person's name and then ask for the immediate superior. The supervisor's response was the same convenient "we are a teaching hospital" speech. I politely explained that there were laws regarding privacy and that I was fully aware that they applied to medical records in all hospitals, including teaching hospitals.

YOU DO HAVE SOME CONTROL, SO EXERCISE IT

We were at a standstill. The supervisor finally said I could send a letter to the hospital stating that I did not want the records removed from the premises and that I only wanted doctors who were directly involved in my daughter's care to have access to them. Aside from not having immediate access to scans that we desperately needed, I was stunned that so many people could be privy to information that I considered private. Our address, phone number, religious affiliation, and genetic testing results were just a few of the pieces of information included in our file, and I assumed they were being held in strict confidence. I wondered why students or physicians we had never met, who had no role in our daughter's care, needed to augment their medical education by leafing through our personal information and then walking off with the scan in violation of the posted rules. If there is information that is unique to one person's medical record that cannot be obtained by attending a lecture, speaking to colleagues, or doing a literature search, then verbal or written permission should be obtained from the patient or his or her family. A patient having ongoing treatment, as Kate was for her cancer, often needs her records on a moment's notice; the staff should be cognizant of this fact.

I wondered what kind of student requests the scans of a patient he has never been involved in treating and then defies university policy by removing them from the medical records department. I envisioned the precious scans tossed into a backpack to be viewed at someone's leisure or to be produced at some opportune moment to impress a superior. A hospital fails both its patients and its students by having lax standards regarding patient privacy and the handling of medical records. There is a small window of opportunity during medical education and training to infuse medical students with respect for privacy and appreciation for the medical record as an invaluable and irreplaceable resource. This opportunity is too often lost and ignored.

DON'T HESITATE TO ASK
FOR RECORDS A SECOND TIME

I had no reason to request medical records again for quite a while. Years later, after Kate's six-week hospitalization for sepsis following a surgical procedure, we were unhappy with her care. We wanted answers explaining how she could have been infected in the operating room with a life-threatening bacterial infection. We were hoping the records would provide us with some insight since the hospital was not forthcoming with answers and was unwilling to investigate the incident to our satisfaction. So once again I phoned the medical records department.

KNOW EXACTLY WHAT YOU WANT AND ASK FOR IT

A recorded message directed me to put my request in writing and to mail it to an address at the university. I sent a very specific request for all records between December 4, 1997 and January 16, 1998 by return receipt mail. It asked for the complete written record, including any notes dictated by physicians. Some doctors, especially in the intensive care unit, use small tape recorders to dictate their patient assessments so their words can then later be transcribed into the written record. These notes may be kept in a separate section of the medical record, and I wanted to specifically include them. I also requested the discharge summary, which is exactly what its name implies—a detailed account of the events of a hospitalization including the initial symptoms and diagnosis, the entire course of treatment, and the condition of the patient at the time of release. They are, in effect, a synopsis of the entire hospitalization process, including admission, diagnosis, and treatment. Discharge summaries are invaluable because they provide an overview of the entire hospital stay and they are usually typed, which makes them much easier for patients to read than the doctor's notoriously bad handwriting.

WAIT AN APPROPRIATE AMOUNT OF TIME; THEN PHONE THE DEPARTMENT IF THE RECORDS DON'T ARRIVE.

I waited for about two weeks before phoning the medical records department. Since I have requested x-rays before, I knew this to be a realistic time frame for a response. I was shocked to hear that they had not received my request, especially since I had proof from the post office to the contrary. Because we live so close to the hospital, however, it was fairly easy to view Kate's medical records in person. (Much later, I would find out what a crucial and fortuitous decision this had been.)

When I arrived at my appointed time, I was given the entire record to view. The medical record was approximately four inches thick and was divided into many sections, which made it difficult to find all the pages for specific dates. I spent hours searching through doctor's notes, surgical notes, lab results, consent forms, and so on, trying to sort out the recent additions from the six-week intensive care stay from the hundreds of other pages.

MAKE COPIES FOR YOURSELF – BUT DON'T EXPECT IT TO BE EASY

Once I felt confident that I knew what I needed copied, I proceeded to ask the staff person to have the sections I had marked with paper clips copied. "Oh, you just do it yourself," he said, pointing to a lone copy machine against the wall. "Just don't take any originals from the record and try not to mix up the pages." The machine took only one page at a time, and every single one had to be fed in by hand. Using a copy service was discouraged since the chart would have to be "sent out." This, of course, would only increase the odds of its being misplaced, and then it could take weeks to receive my copies. Since I was determined to leave with at least some of the records that day, I proceeded to copy as much as time permitted.

Obtaining records may be your right, but it doesn't necessarily have to be easy, efficient, or even affordable, so be patient and persist.

Even in an ideal situation, you will probably need to visit the Medical Records Department of the hospital to mark the sections of the record you need copies of, unless you want the entire record. Once you do this, if you're not in a hurry, the hospital can have an outside company copy the records and mail them you, for a fee.

PORE OVER THE OFFICIAL ACCOUNT OF YOURS, OR YOUR LOVED ONE'S, TREATMENT

Once the ordeal of acquiring the records was behind me, I started to slowly read and digest the "official" account of Kate's hospitalization. *Read* is a relative term here because words, sentences and especially signatures can take several readings to decipher. Finally, we had to construct a timeline and extrapolate some of the names and signatures ourselves. Illegible notes and signatures are common, yet completely indefensible, practices in healthcare delivery systems. When anyone enters information as important as this is, in what functions as legal documents, legibility is absolutely essential.

COMPARE NOTES WITH WHAT YOU *THOUGHT* WAS GOING ON IN YOUR TREATMENT

Much of what medical records contain is factual, objective information. Lab values and test results will be listed numerically or in concise, professional summaries. Conversely, a great deal of the information is subjective and not necessarily based on fact. Progress notes, for instance, written and dictated by physicians, are often brief, one-sided accounts of a patient's treatment; the record and your recollections can differ substantially. Patients have no say in what their physicians enter in this permanent document. They often just assume that they are "on the same page" with their physician. When they're wrong, this can turn out to be a dangerous and even life-threatening supposition. This point was glaringly obvious to us when we read the notes written by the orthopedic surgeon who had failed for five days to diagnose and treat a raging abscess in our daughter's biopsy site. His sparse notes usually consisted of two to three sentences that presented an innocuous picture of her desperate situation.

IF WE HAD KNOWN TO LOOK AT THE MEDICAL RECORD AT THE TIME IT WAS BEING WRITTEN, WE WOULD HAVE IMMEDIATELY REALIZED THAT:

1. We had a right to be worried. Even though we were all looking at the same clinical picture, we found ourselves disagreeing with the doctors about how aggressively they should approach Kate's illness. Only later, when we were able to read her medical records, did my husband and I discover that some of the doctors were actually as alarmed as we were. At the time, the orthopedic surgeon insisted that Kate's biopsy site was not infected and could not be the cause of her life-threatening infection, which hindered the other doctor's inclination to override his wait-and-see attitude and intervene sooner by taking a more proactive approach instead. Even though my husband and I were pressing them for action, the other doctors were extremely reticent to come forward with their own concerns. If we had looked at their notes in the chart, we would have known immediately which doctors shared our opinion, and we could have pressed them to take a stand.

2. The specialists and the ICU staff were not communicating very effectively. This became obvious as we read the first entry by the orthopedic surgeon, the one who was consulted by the pediatric intensivist (ICU physician) the day after her admission to the ICU following a bone biopsy. His entry stated that that a "MRI would be helpful." The subject of a MRI scan first came up two days before the orthopedic consult ever took place. On December 10, 1997, the pediatric intensivist explained that a MRI would give us the answers we needed about the source of Kate's illness, but that it was impossible for a patient to go near a MRI scanner when she was on the type of ventilator that Kate was using to assist her failing lungs. The pediatric intensivist was adamant—he would not risk using a different type of ventilator even for a short time, which made a MRI scan out of the question. If *anyone* in the ICU had read the December 11, 1997 entry written by the infectious

disease physician stating that he "would attempt imaging study (MRI) to see if surgery indicated," or the December 12 entry by the orthopedic surgeon that "an MRI would be helpful," I would have expected them to contact the specialists immediately to clarify that this was not an option, and to aggressively pursue another course of action. Yet, on December 14, the orthopedic specialist again wrote in his notes that "further imaging would be helpful —ultrasound or MRI." Over the course of three days—days that consisted of fever, kidney failure and increased ventilator settings for Kate—the communication and consulting that we assumed was happening at a fever pitch was in a potentially deadly holding pattern.

3. The medical records had an alarming lack of detail and what we considered to be a dangerously one-sided view of the clinical situation. Phrases such as "continue observation," "no significant change," "now responding" and "clinically improved," appeared almost daily and sometimes represented the entire day's entry by that physician. The reality was that her condition was becoming more critical each passing day. There are two problems here. One, the notes did not in any way reflect reality, and Two; the language in the notes was too vague to adequately document the situation. What did the orthopedic surgeon mean by "now responding"? In what specific way was she responding? How could other medical personnel know exactly what the orthopedic surgeon meant by those two words meant without any other information? We'll never know the thought process of the orthopedist because it was never adequately explained in the only document that functions as the official account of a life-threatening ordeal.

When a doctor deems a critically ill patient, or any patient for that matter, "clinically improved," it should be mandatory to include a rationale for their professional judgment in their notes. On December 16, the orthopedic surgeon wrote that Kate was "now moving" her leg, even though the record for that day also shows our daughter receiving a drug to keep her paralyzed so she would not fight the ventilator, Morphine, and a strong sedative. How did a temporarily paralyzed person move her leg? At the time of the surgeon's assessment, Kate was non-responsive and able to make only occasional involuntary movements. But his note made it seem as if she had started to move her leg in some vigorous way and that this was somehow a significant step in her recovery. I was present when the surgeon asked Kate repeatedly if she could feel him pinching her leg. Apparently, her slightest flinch in response to the pain was enough for the surgeon to conclude that this almost nonexistent movement was somehow meaningful, making "continue to follow" a reasonable course of action. When I look back on this time, I have often criticized myself for perhaps wanting and needing to believe that fervent consultations were happening.

4. Every possible avenue was not being explored. In reality, our daughter was not "clinically improved" at all. In fact, she had a sequestered infection in her bone from a biopsy that had been performed five days earlier. When Kate was admitted to the Pediatric Intensive Care Unit, we repeatedly asked if she possibly had an infection from the recent surgery. We were repeatedly told by the infectious disease specialists and several intensivists that the two events were related "in time only" (i.e., it was not a causal relationship) and that they doubted that Kate even had an infection.

In retrospect, it seemed to us that they were unwilling to implicate their hospital in a life-threatening surgical complication. Only later did we read in the record that the admitting diagnosis was right-on-target accurate; it was septic shock (infection). No one would admit to us that they suspected that our daughter had an infection even when they were drawing the blood cultures, starting the antibiotics, or when they summoned an infectious disease specialist. But as Kate's condition worsened throughout the night, who was right and who was wrong lost its place on our priority list. All my husband and I cared about was making sure she woke up alive the next morning.

5. The differential diagnosis contained potential diagnoses that could have been immediately eliminated. When a patient is admitted with an unknown medical condition, physicians will form a "differential diagnosis," where they list all possible diagnosis with the most likely ones at the top. Ask what is included in the differential diagnosis, and write it down. You may be able to add some insight to the confusing clinical picture, which could help later with second opinions or consultations. When I saw that our physicians had included e-coli in their differential diagnosis, I remembered reading that children who were critically ill from e-coli in their bloodstream usually had watery, even bloody, diarrhea. I quickly explained that Kate did not have diarrhea, only soft stools. The physicians still tested for e-coli, but at least they moved it farther down the list.

The differential diagnosis helps physicians keep a broad focus when they don't know the etiology of disease. This is a very good idea. You don't want your team of physicians developing tunnel vision during the diagnostic process and missing valuable clues that could lead to thinking outside the box and discovering an unlikely cause. Patients or their representatives who participate in the initial discussions regarding diagnosis can help clarify the overall clinical picture.

6. Infection (as we had feared) was at the top of the list of suspected culprits. We would have started out working with the doctors as a team instead of feeling like adversaries and being horribly frustrated by the fact that no one seemed to be listening to us. Little did we know that we had all actually reached the same conclusion, but they weren't admitting it. What a shame that we couldn't have operated as a cohesive unit from the first moment and devoted all our energies to Kate's recovery.

7. We needed a second opinion, one from outside this hospital. The
    observations being offered to us at the time came from orthopedic
    residents at the medical center and close colleagues of the ortho-
    pedic surgeon whose authority we were questioning. Of course,
    these people had good reason to be less that forthcoming with us.
    In hindsight, we realized that those people were in the unenviable
    position of possibly disagreeing with a superior. This kind of situ-
    ation can jeopardize professional relationships with more senior
    staff members.

    The orthopedic surgeon, unfortunately, had backed himself
    into a corner. Initially, he examined our daughter for only a few
    moments. All he did was stride into the room, glance at the still-
    bandaged biopsy site and decree, "This is not an infection!" Once
    he had committed himself to such a strong professional opinion,
    however, there seemed to be no turning back. Imagine the embar-
    rassment and ego bruising at having your hasty diagnosis proven
    wrong in front of your students and peers - by the patient's parents
    no less. In the face of Kate's condition worsening by the minute,
    the surgeon simply tightened his grip on his original diagnosis.
    The only thing that could have been done to thwart his stubborn-
    ness was to obtain a completely objective outside opinion.

8. We were entitled to a second opinion from outside that hospital
    system. Once we finally saw that the surgeon was going to take a
    wait-and-see approach, even as our daughter barely clung to life,
    we tried to arrange for an opinion from a doctor at another hospi-
    tal. This experience taught us that even hospital personnel can be
    unclear about the rules.

    The first physicians we contacted refused because they did
    not have "privileges" at our hospital and were under the impres-
    sion that they would not be allowed to consult at a hospital they
    were not affiliated with. Consequently, we were advised to consult
    other orthopedic surgeons within the medical center. The doctor
    in charge of the PICU later told us that we could have obtained

a second opinion from *any* doctor as long as he or she contacted the university and filled out the required forms. Unfortunately, this particular physician was on vacation at the time; all the other doctors we spoke to were either unaware that this was an option or were unwilling to share it with us. The lesson here is not to ask "if" you can get an outside opinion but "What has to be done in order for me to have a doctor from another institution provide a second opinion?"

9. We would have known what the physicians were committing themselves to in writing. What would we have done differently? We would have asked the entire ICU team to communicate more effectively with the specialists by arranging a meeting with all the consulting physicians. The team members could have related their thoughts, concerns and treatment options directly to each other, in which case the "he said, she said" issue we seemed to encounter on a constant basis would have been resolved immediately. We would also have contacted the Patient Relations Department or the hospital administrator to arrange for a second opinion from outside the hospital. We could have voiced our complaints to the chief of staff or the hospital administrator at the most effective time - *as the problem was unfolding*. We could have asked for another surgeon, who was not a subordinate or friend of the first surgeon, who had the integrity to value a child's life over professional courtesy. Most important, we would have given ourselves options. In any tense or life-threatening situation, you want as many options as you can get.

PUSHING THE ENVELOPE – ASKING FOR MY RIGHTS

Many months after Kate's hospitalization, I began doing research for this book. I phoned the Patient Relations Department at the medical center to find out how they would react to a request to view medical records *as they were being written*. The woman I spoke to was kind and informative; she was slightly surprised by, but ultimately supportive of, my request.

I began by asking her about the hospital's policy on viewi records. "Our policy is that patients have access to medical record.., she answered plainly. Off to a good start. Was there was a policy regarding a patient's right to view the record on a daily basis during the hospitalization? Here she hesitated momentarily, then informed me that the record is a "journal" used by the medical staff; as long as the record was not removed from the nurse's station and would be accessible to the staff at all times, she didn't see why it couldn't be read daily. She suggested that patients ask the Charge Nurse or the Nurse Manager to work out a "plan for access." If they met with any resistance, they should phone the Patient Relations Department to facilitate the request.

I wondered aloud if reviewing records on an ongoing basis was an unusual request. Surprisingly, it was the first time in her career she had ever heard of anyone ask for this. "Most people are not willing to delve into such a task because medical records are so difficult to read with all the terminology and abbreviations." I pointed out that this is where legibility was actually rather critical. It was, she agreed, an ongoing problem with healthcare providers with no easy solution in sight. It appeared that bad handwriting was considered as much a part of the history of medicine as listening for vital signs. However, since most hospitals review records to verify that physicians are entering their progress notes in a timely manner, they could conceivably identify staff members who are not providing legible notes and ask them to change their ways.

If you encounter notes that are impossible to read, be sure to contact the administrator's office to alert them. They are the ones who can track down the doctors and ask them to translate their own scribbling. Doctors who don't comply ought to be contacted by an administrator to insist on their unconditional cooperation. In my opinion, this is such a critical issue that physicians who continue to enter illegible notes should have their ability to admit patients suspended.

A small pocket medical dictionary is an essential tool to aid patients in understanding unfamiliar medical terminology. My local bookstore had several to choose from, some in foreign languages and all for less than seven dollars. Medical records may seem confusing at first, but all this means is that people need resources to help clarify, explain and translate; it does not mean abandoning all hope. Like anything else you do, you will improve quickly once you get a feel for it—the learning curve is not that steep. The most powerful intermediaries for medical records access and interpretation guidance are patient relations representatives, social workers, and hospital administrators.

I decided to test the boundaries even further. Could the patient write a note with her own personal assessment of her condition and include comments on her own progress? Could summaries written by the patient or her representative become a permanent part of the medical record? If there was a difference of opinion between doctor and patient, seeing the patient's perspective in writing might give physicians the insight that our harried medical system usually denies them. The practice might also eliminate much of the "we-must-have-had-a-miscommunication" explanation that is so common. Instead of a one-sided account of a hospitalization, I would like to see a two-way street where patients feel entitled to their share of the road. The representative again said that this was unusual, but it "should not be problematic." Remember, the above situation occurred in 1988. New HIPAA (privacy) rules explicitly allow for patients to review and to amend their medical records. It is not longer up to the hospital to "allow" you access, *it is your right*!

She also advised me that a social worker or nurse manager, in an effort to improve communication, could arrange meetings where the family and physicians can discuss together concerns about the treatment plan. They should be held in a private setting, not in the patient's room, if possible, in order for everyone present to be able to speak freely without stressing the patient. These meetings represent a comprehensive review of the patient's progress and future treatment plan, so they are not just quick updates to be rushed through. A social worker or case manager should be present, too, so you can rely on her expertise to clarify, referee, and translate information in the medical record into terms that you can comprehend.

It is in the best interest of patients to have a durable healthcare power of attorney or healthcare proxy, since this simple document authorizes another person to make decisions for you should you become unable to do so. This document allows your designated representative to have access to your medical records, a right guaranteed by the new HIPAA laws. One down side to the beefed-up privacy laws, however, is that they can make it more difficult for a loved one who does not have Power of Attorney to view records, so take care of this important step now. If you are weak or are under the influence of narcotic pain relievers, you will not be up to the task of monitoring and evaluating your information, so delegate the responsibility to someone you trust. Once you have chosen a healthcare proxy, be sure your family and friends know whom you have chosen so your wishes remain crystal clear. Also, select a backup proxy in case your first choice is unavailable or unable to participate. Remember to update proxies in the event of a separation or a divorce.

An update on my original request for medical records (the one they told me they never received): Two months after I sent in the request, I received a package from the medical record center. They had finally decided to send me my daughter's record. A copy of my original request was included and was stamped as being received the day after I had mailed it. The records I asked for dated December 4, 1997 to January 16, 1998, and I knew, because I had stood in front of a machine for hours copying every page of them, that they were about 250 pages long. Imagine my surprise when this package contained a folder with only 50 pages. Had I not gone in to view them in person, I would never have seen the omission. It would be very easy for anybody else to accept an abbreviated version as a complete document, because how would they know the difference? When you call the Medical Records Department, ask them to check how long your record is so you know what to expect.

Action Steps

- Realize that your state may have laws that allow patients to obtain their medical records. State law may allow you even more access to your information, but it cannot mandate less access than what is required by Federal law.

- Request copies of your records, and keep them all together in a safe and accessible place in your home. Keep track of your medical record number at each institution; it will make it easier to access the records. Be prepared to send written requests and to pay duplication fees.

- Ask to review progress notes as they are being written or delegate this task to an advocate. Document the approximate number of pages so you will know how many to expect if you need to request a copy.

- Ask medical personnel to write legibly, to always include the date and time a note is made, and to sign the records clearly. Ask medical students to write "Medical Student" under their notes so orders will not be implemented without being checked.

- Speak to the Charge Nurse or Nurse Manager to work out a "plan for access" if you wish to view your records on a regular basis.

- If you feel the record is not an accurate reflection of your progress, if there is a disagreement about your care, or if the records contain an error, write a note with an explanation of your side of the story, date and sign it, and ask for it to be included in the records. Keep a copy. Realize that this is a provision of federal law.

- Before going to the hospital to view your records, buy a pocket-sized medical dictionary so you can look up any unfamiliar terms you may find.

- Sign a Durable Healthcare Power of Attorney to allow a specific person to make healthcare decisions for you in case you cannot make them for yourself. This paper authorizes your designated agent to access your medical records. Be sure to give a copy to your physician, and bring several copies to the hospital with you so there are no arguments or confusion in the event of the agent stepping in. Be prepared to sign the hospital's preferred version of a healthcare proxy form, even if you have your own with you.

Chapter Eight

Informed Consent

How to Avoid
Signing Away Your Rights

Informed consent occurs after the physician and patient communicate about the diagnosis and treatment plan. The process involves not only communication, but education. The education I am speaking about here is actually a two-way street. Everyone knows that the patient needs to be informed about what is going to happen to his body. What the reader needs to know is that doctors must obtain information from the patient also. They require, among other things, a complete and truthful medical history (people don't always want to disclose their bad habits like tobacco, alcohol and drug abuse), an accurate account of symptoms (people sometimes either minimize their symptoms in an attempt to alleviate their own anxiety or maximize them for sympathy or attention), and an assessment of how aggressively the patient wants his condition to be treated.

A signed consent form – required for all surgical procedures and for many diagnostic tests–is meant to ensure that the patient has been filled in on all necessary information. However, the informed consent is a process involving much more than a single form with a signature. Aside from representing a moral, ethical, and legal requirement for healthcare providers, it represents a sacred covenant of trust between individuals and healthcare practitioners and helps guarantee that patients receive the highest quality of care. The informed consent requirement was established to recognize and protect a patient's right to be an active participant in each and every aspect of the healthcare decision-making process.

Informed consent is viewed as an unalienable right of medical patients, and it is only recently that patients who feel that they have been denied or misled during this process have taken their grievances to court. The case of *Johnson v. Kokemoor* illustrates its importance and brings to light the tragic consequences that occur when someone doesn't know what specific questions to ask before signing on the dotted line.

The plaintiff, Donna Johnson, brought an action against Richard Kokemoor, M.D., alleging that he failed to obtain her informed consent prior to a major surgical procedure. Johnson had already seen her primary care physician with a complaint of ongoing headaches. She was referred to Dr. Kokemoor, a neurosurgeon, who diagnosed a brain aneurysm and performed surgery to repair it on October 1990.

In this case, the surgical procedure itself was a success. However, the patient suffered a horrific adverse event afterward, which left her an incomplete quadriplegic. She is still unable to walk, control her bowels or bladder, and her vision, speech and coordination are all partially impaired. During the court case, her attorneys argued that Dr. Kokemoor overstated the need for surgery and was not forthcoming about his level of expertise with this specific surgical procedure. When the patient asked him how many of these surgeries he had done, she contends that he replied "several." When she pressed him to elaborate more on the number of surgeries, he allegedly replied "dozens" and "lots of times."

The reality was that Dr. Kokemoor had operated on this specific type of aneurysm only twice, and in both cases the defects were smaller and less complicated. He admitted at trial that he had advised Ms. Johnson that the risk of death or serious impairment following this type of surgery was 2 percent, but that her odds were higher due to the location of her defect, but he was unable to give her an accurate number about the increased risk.

Dr. Kokemoor also testified that he was not, and had never been, board-certified in neurosurgery. Ms. Johnson's experts testified that the true risk of death or serious complications from her type of surgery was closer to 11 percent and, even more alarming, that surgery performed by a neurosurgeon inexperienced with this type of delicate surgery could potentially raise the risk to between 20 and 30 percent.

Another issue brought to light during the trial was the expectation that a physician would refer a patient suffering from a rare or unusual condition to the surgeon with the most experience and to a tertiary care center (that is, a major medical center that can provide the highest level of intensive care). In fact, Ms. Johnson was only 90 miles from the Mayo Clinic and may have been better served by its expertise and resources. The Supreme Court of the State of Wisconsin upheld the original verdict for the plaintiff, thereby supporting her assertion that physicians have a duty to inform patients that they may actually receive better care somewhere else, before they consent to being treated locally.

My husband and I are aware of such issues because our daughter had a procedure done that was tacked on at the end of another surgery; we never consented to the additional work. The surgery that we had signed off on was on her knee, and we had actually pushed the physician to do it because we suspected that there was a raging infection in her original biopsy site. During the incision and drainage procedure, the orthopedic surgeon decided, in the operating room, to "tap" the knee joint by placing a long needle into it to remove fluid for analysis by the lab. (We found this out only when he came to see us in the waiting room after surgery.) Several knee taps had already been done in the days preceding this surgery; they had provided only flawed and conflicting results. Knee taps, unfortunately, are not a conclusive test when used to diagnose an infection that lies deep in the bone, and the proof is that even though the knee taps done by the orthopedic surgeon indicated an improvement because the white blood cell count in the fluid extracted from her knee joint was slightly lower, the reality was that Kate's *overall* health was deteriorating rapidly. The white count in her bloodstream was actually high as the result of a growing infection.

The surgery that day confirmed our fears; there was, indeed, a raging infection in Kate's original biopsy site. It also confirmed our belief that Kate did not need another invasive knee tap. The surgeon's defense, when questioned later, was that no harm had been done to the patient. Perhaps, but certainly harm had been done in the doctor/patient relationship, for now we had absolutely no trust in him. Other physicians we consulted told us that his reason for performing the procedure in spite of our wishes might have been a wish to exonerate himself. He knew that his original diagnosis and treatment had been wrong, and he was trying to validate his erroneous decisions by showing that the white cell count had been decreasing, even on the day of surgery.

My husband and I eventually filed a complaint to the Medical Board of California and communicated our displeasure about the knee tap we had not consented to. We thought that certainly there had been a lack of informed consent in this case. But after several months of letters and phone calls, the Board informed us that by signing the "broad" consent form in the first place, we had virtually eliminated many of our rights. According to the Board, the form was "generalized enough" to allow the orthopedist to perform alternative procedures as he saw fit. We were shocked at the news. What choice did we have other than to sign the general form? The hospital hadn't exactly offered us an array of forms and then asked us to choose. For the Medical Board, however, it was the end of the story. It would not so much as look into the issue, and it immediately closed our complaint.

Rushed Signing of Consent Forms

One of the biggest problem-causers is time. Too often, patients are denied a reasonable amount of time to process important information or to ask questions before a consent form and a pen are thrust upon them. I have seen patients asked to sign consent forms they have seen for the first time while they anxiously waited in a "pre-op" area. They are distracted and preoccupied and facing their own mortality. It is not fair to expect people to sign something of significance when they are this fearful or nervous, have no access to their reading glasses, or when they're groggy after being given narcotic pre-operative medications. Recall the wrong site surgery incident discussed in Chapter Four where one poor man had the wrong testicle removed after he signed a consent form without reading it and without wearing his glasses. This is not informed consent; it is "impaired consent," and it will always be a possibility if we don't change our rushed, last-minute medical consent process.

Action Steps

- During the office meeting with the doctor who is planning to perform a procedure on you, ask right then to peruse the consent form. After that discussion, you *must* read and sign the form (with any alterations), or the doctor won't proceed.

- At the hospital, you will have another consent form placed in front of you. Be just as vigilant in signing this one as you were with the form at your doctor's office. If you haven't been able to meet with the surgeon prior to the surgery, or if you need to speak with her again to address a valid concern, have the staff contact the doctor before you sign the form.

- Communicate to any nurse or doctor who asks you to sign a consent form that you don't consider this be a meaningless formality; you take the process very seriously and intend to be fully involved in every way. It may not do anything for you personally, but it does serve the greater good. It lets the medical community know that it is dealing with a growing population of educated patients.

- Let healthcare professionals know that you will sign forms *only* after all your questions have been answered and you feel certain that you possess all the information you need.

LACK OF "INFORMED" CONSENT

When patients are asked to give their "okay" for an invasive procedure to be done to their body, it necessitates full disclosure of facts, risks and concerns. A proper informed consent process addresses several subjects that require detailed discussion. The doctor should fully explain the diagnosis, the reasons that treatment is needed, the risks and the benefits of the procedure, any reasonable alternatives to the procedure, and the risks and benefits of providing no treatment at all. Patients are largely unaware that true informed consent is obtained by the doctor *who will actually be performing the procedure* after he or she has a meaningful discussion with the patient or his advocate. Few patients realize this point: medical ethics dictate that the informed consent process *cannot* be delegated to other staff members. What is amazing is that precisely the opposite practice is actually standard operating procedure in most institutions: the obtaining of consent is often delegated to a subordinate. As a result, patients may find themselves agreeing to procedures they do not fully understand (because the person handing them the form does not have all the information) and/or to having an unknown doctor actually perform their surgery (see ghost surgery). Once you are aware of these risks, you will never take this all-important step lightly again. The signing of a consent form should represent the culmination of a communication process that requires both time and skill on the part of the practitioner. It becomes crystal clear if you realize that, in medicine, the words "informed consent" represent a verb and not a noun. They are not a "thing," but an action.

Action Steps

- If necessary, be willing to change the form to suit your own needs, using the guidelines in the next section.

- Insist on meeting in person with your doctors to have procedures explained to you before you sign anything. This includes the anesthesiologist who will be sedating you. In order to be as informed as possible about what you're letting yourself in for in the operating room, do your research ahead of time. Thanks to the Internet, this has become significantly easier than it used to be. A good starting point is the doctor-designed Web Site www.yoursurgery.com which offers easy-to-comprehend specifics in combination with state-of-the-art animation to inform patients about their surgeries. You can quickly locate the type of procedure being performed on you, print up the notes, and use them to formulate questions to be presented to your surgeon long before you ever enter the hospital. The site offers the following: step-by-step explanations of procedures in terms that a layperson can understand, illustrations of what will be done in surgery, and information on possible complications and expected recovery times.

- Don't be shy about reminding medical personnel that you are aware of the AMA's policy on informed consent. Go ahead and quote the American Medical Association by stating that you know that physicians have an "ethical and legal" requirement to obtain consent personally, after a discussion in which all your questions have been answered.

- Pay close attention to the following action steps for detailed information about parts of a consent form you may want to alter. The bold words and phrases represent alterations you may want to consider.

CONSENT FORMS

Most standardized consent forms used by physicians and hospitals contain similar language. Here's what to look for.

Action Steps

- Look carefully at the "Terms and Conditions of Service" or admitting form which usually states something like "Attending physicians may be assisted by medical students, interns, residents and postgraduate fellows during the care of each patient. The patient agrees to treatment by these persons while under the direction or supervision of the attending physician." Know what you are signing! Do you really consent to care by a medical student who does not have a license yet to practice medicine? What "direction" is the attending physician giving? "Direction" is not necessarily synonymous with "supervision." When a physician is directing, he only has to be accessible for advice and questions. When supervising, he should be physically present and personally overseeing the proceedings. While I do not recommend that patients refuse all outright care by medical residents, I would suggest that you not give away blanket permission for inexperienced or unsupervised medical personnel to take charge of your health care when a lot is at stake. Your attending physician will not always be readily available. It is a given that portions of your care are going to be delegated to interns or residents. Residents will often be writing orders and making healthcare decisions, sometimes behind the scenes. However, you can make sure that you meet the individuals who will be caring for you and be informed about their levels of expertise to judge whether they are competent to treat your condition. It is the *patient* who decides who is a good fit in their healthcare team, even in a teaching institution.

• Patients don't know this, but they can easily alter many salient features of medical admitting and consent forms. Forms can be changed by patients to read: "Patient agrees to treatment by interns and residents on an individual basis through an informed consent process. Patient expects such persons to be under the ***direct*** and ***daily*** supervision of attending physicians." Remember to initial any changes.

• The sentence above the signature line can be changed to state: "I have read the above and agree to the conditions stated ***with alterations***." Again, initial this statement.

• Pay very close attention to "Authorization for Surgery" forms. If left unaltered, they could be a problem because the wording can turn your signature into an open agreement for almost anyone to participate in your surgery. The form will contain wording such as: "I authorize_____, M.D., and associates to perform the following operation(s) or procedure(s)," or something like "I authorize _____ M.D. and other physicians that he/she may designate to perform surgery." This alters specific consent into a "broad" or "blanket" consent because of several key words: "*and associates*" and "*other physicians*." The physicians and attorneys I consulted acknowledged that these words significantly change the meaning and parameters of the consent form in ways that few patients understand. Most people certainly do not intend to authorize "associates" or "other physicians" to perform their surgery without knowing who they are or what their training, experience or level of participation is. But this is exactly what they are doing when they sign to a typical consent form without making any changes. And remember, medical interns and residents are physicians! Be vigilant about signing your rights away, albeit unintentionally. Patients who want the expertise of a particular surgeon should cross out the "associates" or "other physicians" wording on the form and fill in the blank line with their physician's name prefaced by the word "only." For example, "I authorize *only* Doctor John Smith to perform the following operation(s) or procedure(s) as the *responsible surgeon.*" If you encounter any resistance from the hospital about linking your consent to a particular surgeon, it could be an indication that the physician you expected to perform surgery on you has delegated you to one of his residents.

- Ask if your surgeon will be using the services of an assistant surgeon and insist that his or her name be listed on the consent form. The Operative Report is an especially important document because it tells you who actually performed the majority of your surgery. It is a written narrative report completed at the end of each surgical procedure and added to the patient's medical record. Besides the lead surgeon, other participants will be referred to as "assistant surgeons" or they may only be identified by the heading "dictated by," meaning that they were present for and knowledgeable enough about the surgery to dictate the operative report. The assistant surgeon is often the person who is given the job of dictating the operative report. A simple, non-confrontational way to be sure that the surgeon of your choosing will be at the helm is to ask, "When I request a copy of the Operative Report, will I see your name listed as the responsible surgeon? Will you actually be performing the substantive part of my surgery?"

- Some surgical consent forms contain the sentences, "The campuses at XXX Medical Center are teaching hospitals. Consequently, my physician/surgeon may be observed/assisted by residents, interns, students or other allied healthcare professionals." What types of professionals are included in the category "other allied healthcare professional"? This title may sound impressive, but you would be surprised to know that it can include sales representatives, accreditation evaluators, or even members of the media. If you sign an unaltered consent form containing this sentence, you may give up the right to know who will be present in the room during your surgery.

A 1996 survey conducted by the independent non-profit health services research agency, ECRI Institute, showed that 95 percent of hospitals responding to their survey allowed non-surgical staff in the operating room during surgery. Only 53 percent of responding hospitals required patients to consent to it, and only 4 percent actually documented why the outsiders were in the OR in the first place and what activities they participated in. Legally, patients do not have to be informed or give their consent for outsiders to be present in the operating room during surgery. Remember the tragic case of Lisa Smart, mentioned in the introduction to this book. The 30-year-old was admitted to Beth Israel Hospital for routine uterine fibroid surgery and died from an overload of saline solution. The surgeons were trying out a new instrument during the surgery, one they were not properly trained on or authorized to use at the hospital in question, and they needed the medical equipment salesman in the operating room to explain to them how to use the device. The new machine, which ironically had been developed to make fibroid surgery easier and safer, used saline to expand the uterus so that benign tumors would be easier to locate and remove. Allegedly, the salesman operated the controls of the machine while talking the surgeons through the procedure. This means that the surgeons were so unfamiliar with the equipment that the sales representative actually participated in the procedure.

This line of the consent form may be modified to read: "My physician/surgeon may be observed/assisted by others *if their identity, credentials, and experience are explained to me and my informed consent is obtained for any involvement beyond observation.*"

Surgical consent forms often state something to the effect of, "During surgery, additional procedures may be carried out as considered necessary for my well-being by my physician or surgeon for conditions *not known* at the time the operation commenced." This is the specific part of the consent form that caused the California Medical Board to consider it "broad" and that "would allow for other procedures" to be done. It seems that if you sign this as is, you will have no right to complain later when an unexpected procedure is performed. My own experience with the California Medical Board tells me that patients are almost powerless to fight these consent issues *after* the fact. The wording as stated above allows a doctor to perform *additional* procedures, but with two clearly stated restrictions: one, the procedure must be necessary for the patient's wellbeing; and two, it must be performed as the result of conditions *not known* at the start of the surgery.

When I originally read this section, I was under the impression that it was there to benefit patients, that it offered us an added measure of protection against things being done without our knowledge. Procedures would be added only if a patient was in dire need, perhaps even a life or death circumstance. And certainly, additional intervention would only be undertaken if the doctor encountered an unexpected situation that necessitated an immediate emergency decision to save a patient's life. In reality, medical boards, including California's, the medical community, and the American legal system, view this one sentence as a broad, open-ended authorization that provides the surgeon great latitude while in the OR. Usually, doctors only do what they agreed to, but sometimes more may be done than the patient ever realized was possible.

As they are now written, these forms may allow virtually any student, doctor, or unknown "associate" to operate on a patient and to perform additional procedures without the patient's knowledge or consent. This line can be changed to state, "Additional procedures may *not* be carried out unless my designated medical representative gives his or her consent while I am under anesthesia or unless there is a life-threatening medical emergency."

The line on a consent form above the patient signature area can always be altered to say, "My signature is my acknowledgement that I have read, understood, and agreed to the above *with alterations*." Be sure to initial all changes. Patients can easily and legally customize their consent form by lining out words, adding their own words, initialing any changes, and, most important, informing the staff that they *have made changes*. This is important because alterations to a consent form are effective only if the hospital staff is aware of them. Then it can facilitate and implement any necessary changes in their staffing or their scheduling caused by your alterations. Be sure you receive a clear, readable copy of your consent form and keep it for future reference. A good pre-operative discussion with your physician will alert him or her ahead of time to your specific wishes. If you prefer not to have a student or resident perform your surgery, tell your surgeon as soon as possible. The surgery schedule at a hospital is usually very tight, and believe it or not, the surgeon that you expect to be performing your entire procedure may actually be scheduled in another room concurrently. His intention may be to "oversee" your surgery from a distance. Without advance notice, the hospital might not be able to adjust the operating room schedule to let your physician be present for all aspects of your surgery.

It is entirely possible that a hospital will find your alterations to a consent form unusual, but never forget that you are allowed to do it; it can end up being the impetus for meaningful communication between you and your doctor.

Ghost Surgery

The American College of Surgeons lists in its statements on principles of patient care the following standard for surgeons:

"The surgeon may delegate part of the operation to associates or residents under his or her personal direction, because modern surgery

is often a team effort. If a resident is to perform the operation and is to provide the continuing care of a patient under the general supervision of the attending physician, the patient should have prior knowledge. However, the surgeon's personal responsibility must not be delegated or evaded. It is proper for the responsible surgeon to delegate the performance of part of a given operation to assistants, provided the surgeon is an active participant throughout the key components of the operation. . . . It is unethical to mislead a patient as to the identity of the doctor who performs the operation."

Modern-day medical care is always a team effort. There will always be a whole cast of characters, but the American College of Surgeons makes it clear that while delegating is allowed, it must not be done without the patient's knowledge. Unfortunately, all too often, surgeries are performed by someone other than the doctor that the patient is expecting. "Ghost surgery," as this phenomenon is referred to, occurs when the doctor whom the patient knows and expects to perform the procedure either does not actually perform the surgery at all, performs only part of it, or "monitors" from a distance while she is operating on another patient in another room. In short, the captain whom the patient rightly assumes is the steering the ship —isn't.

Patients are virtually oblivious to this practice; they assume that the doctor listed on their consent form will naturally be the one to operate on them. Not always. A standard consent form signed without any alterations by the patient, automatically allows substitutions of surgical personnel, unless the patient makes it clear that he or she simply won't accept it.

My family had an experience with ghost surgery that still angers us to this day. In January 1998, the oncologists wanted to rule out a possible metastasis of bone cancer to our daughter's other leg. Kate was scheduled for a biopsy on her left femur, and we were immediately referred to a particular surgeon because he was the most experienced with pediatric bone tumors. After the biopsy was completed, the doctor appeared in the doorway of the surgical waiting area. He was dressed in scrubs, and his hair and shoes were dressed in the protective paper coverings from the OR. As he held up a specimen container with a small piece of bone floating in a clear preservative solution, he assured us that "this is not cancer. I know what osteosarcoma looks like, and I don't feel that this is what this is." Months later, when we looked through the medical records and saw the Operative Report from the biopsy, we were alarmed to see that it did not contain our surgeon's name, but two unfamiliar names and signatures. Surely, the surgeon who had come out of the OR wearing scrubs and holding the piece of my daughter's bone was the one who had performed the surgery. How else could we have interpreted his presence? What we found was that the experienced surgeon who was listed on the consent form did not actively participate in the surgery and two residents had cut into my child. When I looked back at the form, the two words "and associates" fairly jumped off the page.

The hospital, the Medical Board of California, and several attorneys we spoke to said that since we had signed a "blanket" consent form, we had given our permission for any associates of the surgeon's choosing to perform the operation on our child. Some states have enacted laws to protect the patient's right to give his consent to one individual surgeon only, and they have allowed lawsuits to proceed when patients complained that they weren't informed about a substitution in the surgical schedule. But this is the exception rather than the norm, so don't expect any law to completely protect your right to determine who touches your body. A patient who wants the skill of a particular surgeon needs to clarify her request with the doctor in advance and alter the consent form to state that Doctor X will be present for, and perform, the substantive part of the surgery.

Another practice that is misunderstood is that of monitoring surgery from a distance. People assume that any physician who will be "monitoring surgery" will be physically in the same room as them, looking over someone's shoulder right up until the suturing is completed. However, you should know that doctors may use a much broader definition of "monitoring" than you or I. Some doctors may be comfortable operating in one OR and "monitoring" a second surgery next door; it may even be permissible to leave the surgical area altogether and stay in touch by cell phone or pager. This whole practice certainly seems questionable and I doubt that very many patients would feel secure if their doctor left the operating suite for any length of time during their surgery. Recently, lawsuits have been brought against physicians who actually left hospitals and were on their way home while patients were still in the operating room. All components of surgical procedures are important, even the suturing to close the incision. The moment to be sure that this won't happen to you is when you sign the consent form.

Action Steps

- Inquire into the identities and experience levels of all individuals who will participate in your surgery.

- Have a frank discussion with your physician to lay out your expectations; you want him or her to be present for, and personally direct, all aspects of the surgery.

- Ask outright if a resident will be performing any part of your surgery, what the experience level of that resident is, and how much direct supervision will be involved.

- If you don't want residents in charge during your surgery, let your surgeon know that you routinely request a copy of the Operative Report and that you are counting on seeing him/ her listed as the "responsible surgeon" and not as the "assistant surgeon."

The Coexistence of Education and Patient Care

Does all of this mean that patients should never allow an intern or resident to use their surgery as a teaching opportunity? If this were to happen, doctors would never acquire the needed hands-on surgical experience they require to become certified. Let's not forget that not only do today's patients need quality medical care, so will their children and grandchildren. Consequently, patients must accept the practical need to have students learn on real, live people. On the other hand, physicians should be forthcoming about this practice and be completely honest with their patients. If there were true transparency, and patients felt assured that their safety was the paramount goal even when they're being used to teach students, many would willingly agree to participation by residents, thus eliminating the need for duplicity.

All the patients I treated while I was in dental school knew that the people attending to them almost exclusively were dental students. A certain number of patients came to the dental school because it accepted government subsidized insurance, but many others had private insurance and could have had their dental work completed elsewhere. The dental school offered slightly reduced fees, which also appealed to quite a few. While some patients clearly enjoyed or needed the savings, others were simply proud that they were helping to train the next generation of dental professionals. So they were, in a way, making a contribution to communal healthcare. Our patients knew that they were receiving quality, state-of-the-art care in a safe environment that was closely supervised by experienced dentists and perhaps even dental care that was superior to what one could receive by a mediocre practitioner in his own office.

My experiences tell me that many patients would agree to have an intern or resident perform some of their surgery if a few basic criteria were met. They include:

1. Being told in advance that there will be another participant in the surgery and being asked for their consent.

2. Knowing the identity and training level of the interns or residents and meeting them in advance.

3. Being informed about how much responsibility will be delegated to these assistants.

4. Knowing if the attending physician will be physically present and directly supervise the entire surgery, or if he will be the one to complete the main portion of the procedure while others are allowed to finish. Will he be working in another operating room on another patient and supervise indirectly from a distance?

Of course, patients will make different decisions based on how much they are told prior to surgery. Hospitals may fear that teaching opportunities will be reduced as a result of telling the whole truth, but this is no excuse for not informing patients that their surgery will be a team effort. To keep this train on the tracks, then, physicians simply have to take the time to convey their trust and confidence in the abilities of their residents, explain the importance of giving interns and residents opportunities to learn, and explain the level of participation by both the attending and the residents. Continued involvement by the residents *after* the surgery will make patients feel even more at ease and comfortable with this teaching system. In addition, intensified efforts to improve communication, coupled with genuine respect for patients, will result in an acceptable level of compromise for both patients and doctors. There must be no hidden participants, no ambiguous wording on misleading consent forms, and no misunderstandings or violations of trust due to a lack of communication between patients and their doctors. Medical education can have a powerful role in patient care when the patient's right to informed consent is respected.

Chapter Nine

Your Rights And Responsibilities

The first Patients' Bill of Rights was adopted by the American Hospital Association in 1973 and was expected to improve the quality of our healthcare delivery system. This was the first document to address the principle of patients' rights and included general concepts: the right to respectful care, the right to be informed about a diagnosis and prognosis, the right to privacy, and the right to refuse treatment. The ability of patients to fully understand and participate in their medical care was recognized as the foundation of effective healthcare practices.

For thirty years, it has been the era of patient rights, but it wasn't until 1995 that an issue came up to spark the public debate. That is the year when the public reacted to the managed care policy of discharging new mothers within 24 hours of delivery. The deaths of several newborns from a preventable complication such as dehydration – and the publicity from the resulting lawsuits – led to both public outcry and to attention from legislators. In 1996, states began to pass so-called "drive-thru delivery" laws that allowed for a 48-hour stay after childbirth. The public has also called on the legislature to force managed care companies to pay for breast reconstruction after a mastectomy and to limit "drive-thru mastectomy," a practice similar to drive-thru delivery.

Clearly, people wanted the decision-making ability placed back in the hands of doctors and patients and away from managed care organizations. In early 1997, President Clinton appointed the Advisory Commission on Consumer Protection and Quality in the Health Care Industry, and in November of that year, this commission issued its proposal and provided a basis for a federally mandated Patients' Bill of Rights. The Clinton and Bush administrations have not been successful in guaranteeing patients' rights via a federal law.

There are groups that we would expect to share the same healthcare goals; unfortunately, they have been at odds over the adoption of an effective and enforceable Patients' Bill of Rights. Hospitals, insurance companies, physicians, the American Medical Association, nursing organizations and patient advocacy groups all strive for a cured, healthy, and comforted patient. But these groups seem to pull in opposite directions when the content of a Patients' Bill of Rights is debated because each has its own competing agenda. The situation is especially problematic when lobbyists and legislators are added to the equation. The only entity, it would seem, with relatively little input to the Patients' Bill of Rights is patients—the very group the bill is designed to protect.

While a national Patients' Bill of Rights is vital, however, it will never function at its full capacity if the public is uninformed and uninvolved. People who are unfamiliar with their rights won't be able to exercise them when they are under the stress of being ill and/or hospitalized. As the public awaits a federal mandate, they still have many rights on the books right now that they can insist upon. This chapter will simplify the concept of patients' rights by using the following categories:

1. Diagnosis and Treatment Information

2. Informed Decisions and Informed Consent

3. Privacy and Confidentiality

4. Access to Medical Records

5. To Be Informed about General Hospital Policy and the Complaint Process

6. To Be Informed about All Treatment Options Including the Right to Refuse Treatment

7. To Know the Names, Credentials, and Experience Levels of All Staff Members

8. To Know Financial Information in Advance

9. To Receive Considerate, Respectful and Effective Care

10. Other Rights You Must Insist Upon

1. Diagnosis and Treatment Information

*All information needs to be in language
that the patient can understand.*

Ask medical personnel to speak slowly, clearly, and in lay terms. If patients allow staff members to speak above their level of comprehension, the staff will assume that this is acceptable and will continue to do so. Patients should have a friend or relative with them when communicating with healthcare providers and take notes to refer to later.

Ask for the complete name of your diagnosis.

Sometimes doctors gloss over the technical name of a disease or illness because they're talking to a lay person, and they don't expect him to understand. The patient walks away with a vague notion of what's wrong with him, but not the official term. Without that term, information gathering will be greatly hindered because it is the key to gathering sufficient data from the Internet and other sources. Now the patient does not have enough ammunition even to ask informed questions or make intelligent co-decisions with his physician. Patients often come away from a doctor's meeting shell-shocked. They might remember only being told they have "lung cancer." After that, they have no recollection of what was said about the specific cell type or the exact name of their disease. Yet they need this information to understand the severity of their condition and to participate in their treatment and recovery. A patient could end up spending hours looking up the general term "lung cancer" on the Internet. However, if he can type in "adenocarcinoma," he will be quickly directed to this specific type of cancer; all subsequent research will be easier and more efficient. Write down the complete name of your diagnosis and be sure that you have the correct spelling. If you don't have the presence of mind to ask during the office visit, call the next day after you've emerged from your numb state. When there is a lot of technical information, you can ask the doctor's office to fax it to you.

If a biopsy is involved, you can find out
if a second pathologist reviewed the slides.

Errors in biopsies are rare, but they do happen. Patients should ask to have a second pathologist review their slides. Some institutions have a policy of always double-checking biopsy slides, but patients will not know for sure unless they ask. They can also request a duplicate of the slide and find a second pathologist via another doctor or institution. A second review should be in writing and include the complete diagnosis and signature of the pathologist. Request copies of any pathology report.

Patients are entitled to know the risks
associated with any treatment.

They need to know the risks of all possible complications and the possibility of death associated with a course of treatment. What are the chances of serious complications, infection, or disability? Is there anything that can be done to lower these risks?

Patients are entitled to know their prognosis.

They have the right to as much information as they desire about their prognosis. What is the probability of a successful outcome? What is the physician's experience with their type of disease or illness and how effective has he been? Are there other doctors their physician can consult with who are experts on their condition? Is there anything patients themselves can do to improve their prognosis?

Patients are entitled to have their
course of treatment explained to them.

Before someone can make an informed decision about her treatment plan, she must know what the treatment will involve. How long is it expected to take? What could cause a delay? What can she expect to feel like while treatment is occurring? Will she be able to work? Will it leave her immune system impaired? How many blood draws and/or doctor visits should she expect per week? Will she have to travel to a special facility, perhaps in another city, for certain kinds of treatment?

Patients are entitled to know about
any relevant research protocols.

Will the doctor check to see if any current research protocols or clinical trials are appropriate to include in the patient's care? Does her doctor keep up with the National Cancer Institute listing of clinical trials? If not, she can pursue this option on her own by registering on the NCI Web Site for automatic e-mail alerts for any new clinical trials involving her diagnosis.

*Patients are entitled to a second opinion at any time
during their diagnosis or treatment.*

Tell your doctor you feel it is your responsibility as an informed patient
to seek a second opinion. All doctors should be accommodating at the
very least, and certainly not surprised or annoyed. (If yours makes
you feel uncomfortable about taking this option, then you have
the wrong doctor.) Ask for a recommendation or contact another
institution, your local medical society, or obtain a personal referral
from a friend or relative. Nurses are often a good source for referrals.
They work with many doctors and see both their clinical expertise
and their bedside manner. Many work at more than one institution
and have knowledge about a number of physicians.

2. Informed Decisions and Informed Consent

*Patients have the right to inform their healthcare provider
about their wishes with an Advance Directive.*

Most patients are able to make informed choices about their illness
and treatment options. This information should be put in writing, in
advance, before they are too sick to express their wishes.

*Patients have the right to have all their questions answered,
in lay terms, until they fully comprehend their treatment.*

This is usually done by the person providing the treatment. Find out
the best way to contact healthcare providers if additional questions
arise, and have an advocate in attendance for all discussions with
them. Expect that a professional will spend as much time as you need
on this process. You certainly shouldn't feel rushed or pressured. It is
not your fault that your physician has a tight schedule that day. If he
is genuinely pressed for time, ask for an opportunity to meet again
when you can continue the discussion.

Patients have the right to proper
procedure when signing a consent form.

The person asking you to sign a consent form should be the one performing the procedure, not an assistant, clerk, or other staff member. Read the form carefully and line out any information that does not apply. Verify that the name of the physician and the name of the procedure are filled in and is correct. Consent forms should never be hastily handed to a patient as they are preparing to begin a procedure or after they have had any pre-op medications.

3. Privacy and Confidentiality

Patients have the right to expect confidentiality
of all health and financial information.

This includes all the details in your record, including your address, your employer, your insurance coverage and ability to pay, and religious beliefs.

Patients have the right to confidentiality in all
discussions, consultations, and examinations.

They should know why particular individuals (such as students or specialists) are present during these meetings and can request that these people leave if they are not comfortable with their attendance.

Patients have the right to know what information about
them is being released and to whom it is being released.

They *must* sign an authorization for the release of their information. This is an area to be cautious about when signing a blanket consent form. Patients need to know the names of the parties who will be receiving the information and the length of time their own consent remains in effect.

Patients have the right to expect privacy during the process of sharing and releasing information. Medical information is often shared between many entities, including insurance carriers and government agencies. This process is now governed by federal guidelines designed to protect patient privacy. Violators who disclose medical information inappropriately may face fines and/or imprisonment.

4. Access to Medical Records

Patients have a legal right to their medical records.
This information is not "owned" by the medical establishment. It is, after all, the patient's data. No one should, therefore, encounter resistance when requesting to see her own medical records, it being implied that she's pilfering something that isn't hers. Federal law has finally recognized this, and access is now a guaranteed right.

Patients are entitled to know a physician's or hospital's policy on the release of medical records and how to request them.
A request for medical records must always be in writing. That much is for sure, but doctors or hospitals may have a specific form for requesting records, or they may accept a written letter directly from a patient. Keep copies of all your requisitions and then expect doctors and hospitals to provide a date and time when the records will be available for review or copy, and any costs you will be expected to pay for the duplication process.

Patients or their representatives have the right to view medical records during hospitalization.
Traditionally, the medical chart has been off-limits to patients. A competent patient (i.e., one who is not mentally impaired), however, is entitled to see that record at a time when it will not be interfering with staff duties. Expect to view the record at the nurse's station where it will stay accessible to staff members.

*Patients have the right to make
additions to their medical records.*

Statements, corrections, and additional information can be added to files. Patients can give a provider or an institution a written statement and ask that it be added to their medical record. Anything that is inaccurate or incomplete should be modified with a written statement from the patient. Such statements will become a permanent part of the medical record, so whatever patients write should be clear, concise and accurate.

*Patients have the right to expect
their medical record to be legible.*

Medical records are not only legal documents that chronicle every aspect of patient care, but also a vital means of communication between healthcare providers. Entries that are illegible compromise care and can make it almost impossible to evaluate its quality at a later date. Hospitals rely heavily on chart review so they can assess quality of service. If charts are incomprehensible or unreadable, the consequences are clear: someone could receive a medication he's allergic to, an unnecessary procedure could be performed, and so on.

Illegible medical records continue to represent a serious, ongoing threat to medical consumers, and they are, unfortunately, a widespread occurrence, as was confirmed by court reporters who were interviewed for this book. They report that some records are so badly written that sometimes a deposition has to be taken for the sole purpose of translating it, with the help of a physician who deciphers his own entries. One court reporter I interviewed estimated that 25 to 30 percent of her medical malpractice depositions included requests for physicians to translate portions of their own illegible notes. During depositions, physicians have even resorted to making "educated guesses" as to what their notes say since they can't read their own writing months later. Patients should tell their providers that they expect them to keep the entries into their medical record usable by making them readable.

5. To Be Informed of General Hospital Policy and the Complaint Process

Patients are entitled to reasonable visitation by loved ones.
Normal visiting hours may not meet everyone's needs, so they should be flexible if you ask the hospital ahead of time. Even those in special areas such as intensive care units have the right to see friends, relatives and colleagues. If visiting hours are completely unsuitable, patients or their representatives can contact Patient Relations or the hospital administrator and make other accommodations.

Patients have the right to have a friend or
relative stay with them 24 hours a day, if necessary.
Parents, especially, sometimes need to stay with their children around the clock. Generally, hospitals recognize this need, but adult patients also have the same requirements at times – to have an advocate stay with them – and this should be respected. Just inform the nursing staff so they can try to make sleeping arrangements.

Patients are entitled to have visits from their children or siblings.
Isolation from family members can have a harmful effect on both patients and their relatives. Because children carry so many viruses and germs, they may need a nurse to take their temperature prior to a visit. (In any case, they should certainly wash their hands before entering a sick person's room.) Children who are not feeling well should avoid the hospital until they have recovered.

Patients have the right to lodge formal complaints
about any aspect of their care.
If they need additional information, the Patient Relations Department

can inform them about the complaint process. Please note that complaints are more effective if they are made in writing.

Patients have the right to know the disposition of their complaint.
Complaints can sometimes be addressed immediately and a solution can be attained. Others may not be resolved until after a patient is discharged. In this event, patients should expect a written response.

6. To Be Informed About All Treatment Options, Including the Right to Refuse Treatment

Patients have the right to a discussion of all treatment options even those not covered by their HMO or other insurance plan.
Patients need a comprehensive treatment consultation of suitable length to evaluate what direction they want to head in. Insurance companies have tried in the past to limit physicians to discussing only those treatment options that their plan will cover, but this practice has been deemed a violation of the integrity of the doctor-patient relationship and is never appropriate.

Patients have the right to refuse treatment.
They are the ultimate decision-makers concerning their healthcare. Even when providers disagree with his choice, it is the patient's right to refuse any part of a treatment plan. Patients wishing to forego any further invasive or heroic interventions should sign a Do Not Resuscitate (DNR) order.

*Patients have the right to supportive care
even if they have refused active treatment.*
Those who have refused active treatment for reasons of their own are still suffering. They may still need quality supportive care for oxygen therapy, complications, or pain management as much as anyone else.

Patients have the right to know their options when
they no longer have to be in the hospital but still need care.
Many patients will reach a point in their illness when hospital care cannot meet their needs because the institution is not set up to provide long-term care or rehabilitation therapy. They are entitled to a realistic assessment of the role a hospital can play in their care, and advice about what to do when that role ends.

7. To Know the Names, Credentials, and Experience Levels of All Staff Members

Patients should expect all staff members to wear
a badge with their full name, picture, and title.
Institutions have strict rules about their employees wearing identification at all times, and you must be sure to read them and keep yourself informed. Knowing the names and titles of the individuals caring for you is essential.

Patients have the right to ask staff members how long they
have been working in their career and at their institution.
It is never intrusive for a patient to inquire about a staff member's work experience when his life is in that person's hands. This is not an insult nor a challenge, but an attempt by the patient to remain an active and interested participant in his own recovery.

Patients have the right to ask how many times an
individual has performed a certain procedure.
Patients are entitled to assess what the provider's expertise is based on the number of procedures performed and on the person's success rate.

Patients have the right to inquire into a staff
member's certification and licensing.
The only information that name badges provide are a person's name and job title. That doesn't always inform you of her real qualifications.

Someone who became a nurse's aide in a different state doesn't necessarily have the same level of training as a person trained in your state, which may have more stringent guidelines. Patients have the right to know the training, skill level, and certification methods for all individuals. In addition, unlicensed personnel can have confusing titles that don't immediately alert patients that they have little training. Don't feel bad about asking, "Are you licensed by the state?" If a staff member doesn't seem up to par with others, you need to be vigilant to make sure he or she knows what she's doing. Don't feel bad about asking that this person perform certain procedures, such as inserting a catheter or an IV line, under the supervision of someone more experienced.

Patients have the right to refuse treatment by medical or nursing students.
If you are unwilling to have a serious injury or complicated illness treated by interns, residents, nursing students, or medical students—even in a "teaching hospital"—you are able to say so. On the admission form, line through the clause that permits the hospital to have part, or all, of your treatment performed by students. Even in a teaching hospital, you have the right to limit your consent regarding treatment by students.

8. To Know Financial Information in Advance

Patients have the right to know if the necessary authorizations are in place prior to treatment.
Doctors and hospitals are responsible for securing any authorizations required by an insurance carrier. If there are any problems or delays in the authorization process, you should be notified since you are the one responsible for payment if a service is denied after the fact.

Patients have the right to know about all payment options.
They should be told what co-payments they are responsible for, when payment is expected, and what payment plans are available.

Patients have the right to know what
will happen if they have no insurance.

Uninsured patients must be told how much responsibility they will have to assume to ensure payment of medical bills. Are there state or federal government services available that will require them to complete forms and/or make appointments for interviews?

9. To Receive Considerate, Respectful and Effective Care

Patients and their representatives have
the right to be treated with respect and dignity.

Their opinions, medical and emotional needs, and decisions should be handled with courtesy and consideration. Patients are paying customers, and they are entrusting the institution with their lives.

Patients have the right to receive efficient and coordinated care.

Everyone needs medical treatment that is managed well and scheduled correctly to minimize unnecessary feelings of invasion and trauma. For example, all blood samples may be able to be drawn at the same time so patients are only poked once.

Patients should expect a high level of communication
between staff members and between staff and patients.

The quality of medical care is dependent upon the ability of the staff to communicate effectively with each other as well as with patients and their families. Staff tends to communicate both verbally and through entries in the medical record. Patients have the right to insist that they consult among each other on a regular basis and before any treatment decisions are made. Patients should expect them all to take enough time to explain procedures and treatment to them.

Patients have the right to expect continuity of care.

The quality of healthcare improves whenever the people who are familiar with the patient's treatment plan are consistently the ones who continue to care for the person. But this is a problem when institutions rotate the assignments of patients to nurses in order to maximize their opportunity to receive training and experience. Patients do have the right to request that staff members who know them remain a part of their team. They can also expect the staff to micromanage the treatment plan so that procedures such as blood draws are coordinated and performed together whenever possible.

Patients and their advocates have the right to participate in their own medical treatment.

They need to be recognized as vital members of the healthcare team and encouraged to participate in the recovery process. If this mindset is lacking in your hospital, you need to be vocal about your intention to participate fully in your care.

10. Other Rights to Insist Upon

The right to have an advocate present for the induction of anesthesia.

The thought of receiving anesthesia is terrifying to many patients, so to relax, they need pre-op medication prior to heading into the operating room. They also feel less anxious if a friend or relative accompanies them. When arrangements are made ahead of time, patients can often have an advocate present in the operating room area and stay with them until they are asleep.

The right to have an advocate present in the recovery room.

Many hospitals are beginning to recognize the need for patients and their loved ones to be together as soon as a patient is awake after a procedure. An advocate who is familiar with the patient can have a great impact in the recovery room setting. The person can help assess pain levels and communicate to recovery room personnel what is needed, and he can help control the kind of agitation that occurs when a patient awakens confused and alone.

The right to effective pain control at all times.
Patients are entitled to know in advance the plan for managing their pain. If the original plan isn't effective, what happens next? Who is authorized to increase or change the medication orders? Will this person be accessible after hours? Is there staff present at all times who will be able to administer these medications?

Now that we have covered your rights, it's time to review the areas where you, as the patient, are accountable.

Patients Have the Responsibility to:

*Be honest and complete about your medical
history and be frank about your vices.*
If you have a gin and tonic and a cigarette every day at five, and the doctor asks if you drink or smoke, don't say no just because you only do it once a day. There is a natural desire for people to cover up their vices, but this is neither the time nor the place to do it. What the doctor doesn't know *can* hurt you. In some cases, it can severely affect your diagnosis and treatment plan. Be careful to relate all information concerning medications (including over-the-counter medications and natural or herbal supplements), past hospitalizations, illnesses, illicit drug use and other high-risk behaviors, as well as your fears to your healthcare providers.

Voice all concerns, doubts and fears.
Patients must express any reservations that come up about accepting, following, or completing a treatment plan. Don't wait until it's too late to do anything about it. Even if you think it's silly or neurotic, say what's on your mind. It could save you a great deal of trouble down the line, and it will certainly improve your relationship with your physician by leveling with her. Often, your fears are without basis, and telling your doctor what they are gives her a chance to allay unnecessary worries so you can relax.

*Ask questions and tell staff members when
you do not understand what is happening.*

If you are confused around what is about to happen to you, when a procedure will take place, why it has to happen, how it will be done, or who will do it, you have to communicate these questions effectively to those entrusted with your care. The anxiety brought on by unanswered questions will not help the recovery process. And there may be times when the answers prompt you to contribute important information of your own.

Be an active participant in your medical care.

You have the responsibility to inform yourself about your condition and to speak up if something doesn't seem right. You might be wrong, but it's better to speak up anyway, if for no other reason than to satisfy yourself that all is well and everyone is on the right track. And don't be afraid to alert staff members if you are unsure about any unexpected changes to your treatment plan or to report errors and complaints to the proper administrator.

Understand what is expected of you as a patient.

You need to know exactly what is expected of you before, during, and after your treatment in order to be a full and complete partner in your recovery. How many office visits and blood draws will be needed? How many x-rays or scans have to be scheduled? How long will visits last? How long will follow-up care last? What will be asked of you?

*Follow the treatment plan or communicate
immediately why you either cannot or will not follow it.*

If you have a problem with time, fear, pain, costs, or how your work schedule will be impacted, you ought to discuss that with the proper parties. Not doing this could seriously influence how much you cooperate and assist with your own treatment plan.

Take responsibility for refusing treatment after making a careful, informed decision.

Don't expect to go back after the fact and blame the hospital if you suffer ill effects from not taking your medicine, not undergoing surgery or chemotherapy, and so on. You cannot, in all conscience, point the finger when you are the one who chose to not follow doctor's orders.

Recognize and meet your financial obligations.

Patients are responsible for the financial cost of their treatment. They are also responsible for providing a healthcare organization with all information needed to process a claim. You must be prepared to work with the hospital to secure payment.

Follow the rules and regulations of a facility.

Hospitals have these rules because they oversee the care of a staggering number of patients, each with a different condition and requirement. It would be chaos if every patient set his or her own agenda. It's important to be considerate and recognize that the needs of a lot of people have to be met by this hospital, not just yours. Sometimes, however, a patient genuinely needs to adjust the rules of a medical institution. If you do, make arrangements through the proper channels and in advance because it gives the staff the time and opportunity to accommodate your needs. You can ensure that your needs are met by making your preferences about private rooms, visitation, meals, and rooming-in policies known to any appropriate staff member.

Provide a copy of your Advance Directive or Do Not Resuscitate order to the hospital.

Patients with an advance directive should have it notarized, and provide the healthcare institution with a written copy to be kept with the medical record. They should keep their own copy of their directive or DNR with their belongings in case the one provided to the hospital is lost. A family member or any other individual who has medical power of attorney should always have a copy of either document readily available.

Chapter Ten

A Review of the Information and Communication Process:

Prerequisites for Becoming a Proactive Patient

To effectively monitor hospitalization, either as a patient or as an advocate for another person, you need to take a proactive approach. It is vital that you begin a thorough information-gathering process about our medical system long before hospitalization or the diagnosis of an illness. (With WebMD and other Internet sites, the public now has a prodigious amount of medical data at their fingertips.) Information, as the saying goes, is power. Why is it more important than ever for patients to collect and share their own information and research with their doctor? Because it empowers them to realize that they are solid members of their own healthcare team. To truly feel this way, they have to be able to field the ball and step up to the plate to bat. They must have a firm hold on what they've learned so they can communicate effectively and offer intelligent, well-researched opinions that matter.

Information also gives patients the skills to manage their symptoms and reduce unnecessary emergency room and physician visits. This is not only good for the patient, but it helps the entire system by keeping costs down—a true win-win situation. Information is now so important that it is considered a form of therapy for patients. It takes some of the mystery out of what's going on, and it lets people comprehend the extent of their condition so they can undertake specific actions needed to manage it. By seeking information as soon as a diagnosis is made, patients place themselves on the right track. There is less opportunity to sink into denial, depression or paralyzing fear. It is always less anxiety-provoking to know what you're up against than to let your imagination run wild. Fear tends to drive thoughts to their most catastrophic conclusions. Working on a plan of action as soon as possible provides a sense of control and accomplishment. Everyone feels better doing something rather than doing nothing at all.

I can think of a number of people who took a proactive approach and benefited from it. One woman read all about lumpectomies versus mastectomies and then was able to ask her surgeon for the former and less invasive approach. I have a patient who is a diabetic. Her doctor had always told her that she didn't need an insulin pump, but she researched it and brought what she learned to her doctor. He agreed that the pump really was the best course for her. Perhaps he would have gotten around to suggesting it sooner or later, but maybe not. Doctors often assume all is well unless the patient speaks up and says, "I think we can do better than this." My own husband is another good example. His father died of a heart attack at a young age, and we have always been aware that John could follow in his footsteps. We read that there were simple blood tests to check for inflammation in the coronary vessels, a potential precursor of heart attacks. If the test came back positive, all that would be needed is a daily dose of aspirin!

John found that his C-reactive protein and homocysteine levels were normal, a fact that relieved us of a great deal of anxiety. While our doctor readily agreed to the test, it wasn't his suggestion.

We are way past the day when we could expect physicians to have every detail of health information on the market stored in their heads or even find it readily in textbooks. In this age of information, patients have so much at their fingertips that they are often able to educate their doctors. I always appreciate it when patients bring news articles or new technologies to my attention, because they have done some of the leg work for me! Making a compilation of information from an array of sources—such as healthcare providers, the Internet, books, magazines, newspapers, television programs, family, friends, professional organizations such as the American Cancer Society or the American Heart Association, online communities and online message boards—will give patients the best chance for catching important facts about their condition. Sharing the weight of the responsibility for obtaining and sharing information will ultimately allow patients to assume confidence in, and control over, their medical care.

The following steps represent ways in which patients can do their legwork ahead of time and have all necessary information at hand:

1. Maintain a medical diary

2. Understand, research, and confirm a diagnosis

3. Obtain and comprehend test results

4. Make the most of your time with your physicians

5. Plan for returning home from the hospital

Maintain a Medical Diary

CURRENT CONDITIONS AND CHRONIC ILLNESSES

Be prepared to give a concise summary of both your current health status (i.e., colds, infections, and temporary back pain) as well as any chronic illnesses (i.e., colitis, ulcers, and arthritis).

PREVIOUS DIAGNOSES

Keep a list of all previous diagnoses, both major and minor, the date of the diagnosis, and the name and contact information for the physician who cared for you. This lets your current doctor consult with the previous provider to see how the person arrived at his or her diagnosis.

MEDICATIONS

Tell your provider about all medications you have taken in the past, are currently taking, and who prescribed them. Include information on dosages and number of times taken per day. A great idea is to keep a small medication record in your wallet at all times. Many doctors' offices can provide one, or you can print one off the Internet. Whenever you see new providers, they can make a quick copy of all pertinent information taken straight off the small card. I love seeing patients come in to my office with these cards for two reasons: one, I know that I am getting a complete and accurate account of all their medications. They don't have to sit there and wrack their brain for an hour to remember what medications caused negative reactions. Two, I immediately know that I am dealing with an educated, cooperative patient who is willing to go the extra mile to keep her doctor informed and to keep her safe. Medication usage is fraught with secrets because patients often adjust dosages, cut back on medications to save money, or start to feel well and don't think that they need as much. Tell your doctor about *all* over-the-counter medications (i.e., Tylenol, ibuprofen, calcium supplements, sleep-aids), since they have active ingredients that may have a negative interaction with prescription medications.

Also inform your physician if you are taking nutritional supplements and herbal or "natural" remedies. These sometimes cause worrisome symptoms in patients or counteract the effects of a prescription. For example, the natural medication St. John's Wort may reduce the effectiveness of birth control pills. Herbal diet medications often contain ingredients that produce an effect on the body; it would be a mistake if that effect were attributed to another cause because the doctor didn't know you were taking it. Some, for instance, stimulate the body and lead to a rapid heart rate or feelings of agitation. A doctor would be less apt to over treat a rapid heartbeat if he knew that the patient had been taking stimulant-type natural diet aids.

ALLERGIES

Keep a record of all allergies, even allergic reactions to simple things like betadine or the adhesive on tape. Note what symptoms appeared and how long they lasted. List any medications used to stop the reaction and the name of the doctor who diagnosed the allergy in case the person needs to be consulted at a later date. And remember, just because you weren't allergic to a medication in the past does not mean that you couldn't be now. Our bodies change all the time. I knew someone who wasn't allergic to poison oak as a boy. As a young man, he went hiking right through a patch of it to impress his friends, who were all very allergic. He overexposed himself, and that evening, he broke out so badly that he had to be taken to the hospital. Just recently, I prescribed a common antibiotic for a patient. He had taken the same medication in the past with no ill effects, but this time he ended up in the emergency room with hives and a restricted airway. After taking some Benadryl and steroids he was able to go home, but it was a harrowing ordeal for all involved.

ALL TREATING PHYSICIANS

Keep a list of all the physicians who have treated you, past and present, and the amount of time you were under their care. However, you don't need the name of the guy who took out your tonsils when you were four years old. It is the doctors from the recent past who must be kept track of. Also include any physician who diagnosed a serious problem because your current doctor may need to consult with him or review his treatment records. Include contact information such as phone numbers, fax numbers, or e-mail addresses.

DATE OF MOST RECENT PHYSICAL EXAM

You should know the date and the results of your last physical exam and record your weight, blood pressure, cholesterol level, and any other pertinent information. The names of all immunizations and the dates you were given them are also vital to have written down so the doctor can determine if you are adequately protected against disease and give you any booster shots or additional doses. Request a copy of all blood and urine test results to keep with your diary. Note the name of the physician who performed the physical and her contact information.

DATES OF HOSPITALIZATION

Make sure you can provide the dates of all hospitalizations, the admitting diagnosis, and the discharge summary of the treatment received. Record the medical record number, even if you think you've memorized it.

THE LOCATION OF X-RAYS AND OTHER TEST RESULTS

Keep a record of all your x-rays, scans, and other studies. The dates of the tests, the name of the institution, and the written report issued after the tests were reviewed should also be part of this record.

COMPLETE DISCLOSURE BY THE PATIENT

We all are guilty of trying to hide our bad habits, but patients must disclose their use of tobacco, alcohol, and drugs. Most people hide the truth because they are worried that the doctor will criticize or judge them. It is in your best interest to admit that you are human, that you have a few vices, or that you may not have told the complete truth or followed all the doctor's orders. For example, you may present with poor wound healing after a surgery. The doctor asks if you have been following recovery recommendations—don't lift heavy objects, don't have a smoke, don't drive your car. Instead of telling a seemingly harmless fib, admit that you've been slipping and sliding so the doctor doesn't grow alarmed and think you have another condition that is causing your wound to heal slowly. He might then order invasive tests to figure out why your healing process is taking so long. By this point, you might feel too far into the little white lie to turn back.

INJURIES AND SURGERIES

You need a record of all injuries that required treatment and every surgical procedure. The complete name of the injury or procedure should be noted, in medical terminology. Include all dates, the name of the treating physician, the length of treatment, and a copy of the operative report and pathology report from all surgeries.

FAMILY MEDICAL HISTORY

If possible, maintain a record of the illnesses of all family members, their age at their death, and their cause of death. There are a whole slew of diseases that tend to run in families, and it can be helpful to your physician to know that your father developed diabetes or that cancer runs on your mother's side. One man I know was diagnosed at an early age with colon cancer. His doctor advised him to have all of his siblings tell their respective physicians immediately and recommended colonoscopies for each one. One sister had just had a sigmoidoscopy a couple of years earlier, so her doctor felt sure that a colonoscopy was not warranted. The brother's doctor, however, kept insisting that every single person had to be checked because this type of colon cancer ran in families. Sure enough, the same sister whose doctor counseled against a colonoscopy was also diagnosed with colon cancer and required immediate surgery. Fortunately, her timely diagnosis spared her the chemotherapy and radiation treatments that her brother had to endure. Your genetic history can prove immensely valuable to your doctor, so ask relatives or look at death certificates to try to ascertain the illnesses and cause of death of as many relatives as you can.

ADJUNCTIVE HEALTHCARE PROVIDERS

Keep a record of all chiropractors, acupuncturists, physical therapists, nutritionists, and any additional providers of health services. Your physician may need to consult with these providers to figure out what injury or illness you were being treated for, and the other providers may have valuable records such as x-rays to share.

INSURANCE INFORMATION

Make sure you have instant access to the name of your insurance carrier, group number, and the phone number and billing address for the insurance company. It's the first thing they ask for, and there's a reason for that. The hospital needs to be sure you're covered and you need to be protected from being denied coverage, at a later date, for certain treatment. Your Social Security number and birth date of the subscriber will also be required. Make a copy of your insurance card and give it to the person who has your medical power of attorney. In an emergency it is handy for a close friend or family member to also have this information so they can complete the registration process at the hospital.

Understand, Research, and Confirm a Diagnosis

UNDERSTANDING THE DIAGNOSTIC PROCESS

Patients can be confused and overwhelmed by the events preceding a definitive diagnosis. In general, the order is as follows:

1. The patient presents with a condition that concerns her enough to seek medical attention.

2. The healthcare provider starts to order tests to gain information about a possible illness.

3. If the results are inconclusive, the patient is referred to a specialist who is more experienced in diagnosing and treating specific conditions.

An evaluation of the symptoms, a physical examination, and initial tests such as blood tests or x-rays will often only give the primary care physician a starting point. Advanced studies such as CT scans, MRI scans, or tissue biopsies will confirm a diagnosis and aid in formulating the treatment plan. Additional tests are usually needed both before and after a diagnosis is determined to aid in treatment planning or to assess the efficacy of a treatment. The diagnostic process can seem unbearably slow to the patient and his family, but just as attorneys won't enter a courtroom until they have all the facts relevant to a case, physicians won't proceed with treatment until they've had time to evaluate all the information from every test and determine its overall significance.

NAME OF CONDITION

As stated in a previous chapter, patients must know and record the complete name, in medical terminology, of their diagnosis. This information is needed to research a diagnosis or to converse with other healthcare professionals.

STAGE

Some medical situations, such as a diagnosis of cancer, will include information on the "stage," or extent, of the disease. Staging is part of the diagnostic process and can help physicians determine a prognosis or odds of healing. It involves evaluating variables such as size, location, the invasiveness of a disease process, and the presence of tumor "markers"(genetic clues to the way a tumor will behave), which are evaluated by both clinical and laboratory data. Staging provides important information that can impact both present and future treatment. Breast cancer is one illness that clearly demonstrates the importance of this step. The treatment plan for it is greatly influenced by whichever stage the person is in. Decisions about whether to do a mastectomy versus a lumpectomy, for instance, about adding radiation therapy or about the need for medications like Tamoxifen to prevent a recurrence of disease – are all affected by information on the stage at which the disease was diagnosed.

IS THERE METASTATIC DISEASE?

After a diagnosis of a malignancy, tests will be performed to determine if metastatic disease (metastases) is present. This term refers to the presence of disease in an area that is different from the primary or initial site of a tumor. This is crucial information because metastatic disease is often more difficult to treat than something that is only local, and usually it requires more aggressive treatment. A finding of it will often lead to revisions in the treatment plan in order to give the patient the greatest chance of beating the disease.

IS THIS A CHRONIC OR AN ACUTE CONDITION?

Patients are often distressed at the time of a diagnosis. They don't even know that they need to ask whether their condition is acute or chronic. If a condition is acute, most likely it will run its course, and the patient will ultimately recover fully and have no residual, permanent effects. A chronic condition, however, may require permanent lifestyle adjustments, life-long use of medications or ongoing testing. If you are diagnosed with a chronic condition, you will want to ask what changes will take place and what extra responsibilities they will place on you. For example, a patient has a pacemaker implanted but doesn't realize he will need to take medications for the rest of his life. The patient may not realize at the time that he will need to see a cardiologist regularly to have the pacemaker tested and adjusted. He might even need more surgery to replace the battery periodically. Of course, knowing that the life-saving device comes with additional responsibility would hardly lead the patient to reject it, but asking a few simple questions will immediately afford him greater comprehension of the realities of his diagnosis. Ultimately, this leads to less stress and confusion at a time when all his energy should be placed on improving his health.

RESEARCHING THE DIAGNOSIS

By now, you probably realize that you must take responsibility for researching your own condition and obtaining your own independent information as a form of quality control. The public is quickly learning that it is not in the nature of modern medicine to allow patients an unlimited amount of time with their physicians. There is no guarantee that they will receive every single pertinent, up-to-date piece of information about their condition. So, in this day and age, a diagnosis is a call to action for the patient and anyone around them who can help gather information. It is a little like the intelligence-gathering process in the military. A potentially threatening situation presents itself, the experts begin to utilize all their known sources of information, and then all involved meet and confer to share data and make a decision. The Internet can be a valuable tool to research a diagnosis, but don't be discouraged if the information seems overwhelming, difficult to understand, or even outdated. Rely on well-known, reputable medical Web Sites including WebMD.com, Mayoclinic.com, Medscape.com, and MedlinePlus.gov. Online message boards or chat rooms may also provide useful information (others with the same condition may have many time-saving and helpful suggestions), but be sure to safeguard your private information. Books are another helpful resource, and typing in the specific condition or a related concept to online bookstores such as Amazon.com can give you instant access to all relevant titles. There are companies and organizations that will, for a fee, research a medical condition and provide a written report with all the current information available. If you are interested in these services, contact:

The Health Resource, Inc.
www.thehealthresource.com
(800) 949-0090 or by email at research@thehealthresource.com.

Or:
Mr. Health Search
www.mrhealthsearch.com at (800) 794-5015;
email moreinfo@mrhealthsearch.com.

CONFIRMING A DIAGNOSIS

An accurate diagnosis is a prerequisite for any appropriate treatment plan, and that is difficult to achieve when there are vague symptoms that could lead doctors to consider a variety of illnesses. Your primary care physician will almost always be aided by other specialists, and they will begin by ordering tests. Only after examining the patient personally, arriving at a consensus on the meaning of all the symptoms and interpreting all the information from tests, does a diagnosis start to take shape. Information often trickles in slowly, however, and may even be contradictory at times; it is not always an easy, straightforward process. Tempting as it is, don't try not to become overzealous and pressure healthcare professionals to rush through the diagnostic process. And certainly, don't let any physician rush *you* through the process.

SECOND OPINIONS

As I have said previously, patients *always* have the right to seek a second opinion. They must trust their instincts and not dismiss their doubts because the "doctors must know what they're doing." Only rarely is time so critical that it impossible to take a few days, or even a few weeks, to contemplate all one's options and to arrange to ask for another doctor's advice. A compilation of irrefutable proof is vital, even thought it is potentially time-consuming, and both patients and physicians must be confident about the diagnosis before embarking on a treatment plan. By all means, for any serious medical condition, do not hesitate to seek a second opinion. See Chapter Five for a detailed discussion.

Obtain and Comprehend Test Results

What tests are being ordered, and why are they needed?

Expect a discussion with your physician listing the tests being ordered and explaining why they're necessary. Certain tests are absolutely imperative for formulating a diagnosis, yet the patient doesn't always see the big picture. Why does he question their importance? Because we have not forgotten the days when physicians tested for everything under the sun just to be sure people couldn't turn around and sue them for not covering all the bases. Some patients didn't mind the good old days. After all, "the more tests, the better, right? And the insurance company is paying for them anyway, so why not be sure." Nowadays, we all know about the downside of too many tests: risks of over-radiation, unnecessary fears caused by looking "too hard for something wrong," and the invasiveness of biopsies that are brought about because false-positive results. Of course, we are also no longer naïve about insurance costs being passed along to us in the form of higher premiums.

Testing, quite simply, is no fun. It is sometimes painful and risky, and it certainly provokes a good deal of anxiety. Make certain you are informed about the purpose of each test and understand its diagnostic value in your treatment. Test results are like pieces of a puzzle in which many bits of information need to be fit together in order to complete the picture. Ask your doctor what specific facts you will receive from this test, so your expectations will stay realistic. For example, a patient might be counting down every minute as he waits for a definitive diagnosis about whether he has cancer without realizing that this test won't give him the doctor all the information needed to make that diagnosis.

What are the risks, side effects and recovery time?

You are entitled to a discussion with your physician about the risks involved in every diagnostic procedure. The discussion should include information about side effects, any pain that will be suffered afterwards and how it will be managed, and the expected recovery period. Many patients who consent to a spinal tap, for instance, are not aware that they could have an excruciating headache afterwards requiring narcotic pain relief. It is not uncommon for patients who have had a surgical procedure to be unprepared for the amount of pain it engenders, for the recovery time to drag on a lot longer than they thought it would, and for tubes and drains to be hanging out of their body for days after surgery. People who have biopsies in sensitive areas or near certain muscle groups are unexpectedly stiff, sore, and unable to function well for longer than they expected. All of this uncertainty could be avoided if their doctors had discussed the situation with them and told them what to anticipate or if the patient had known to ask more detailed questions.

Remember, consent to proceed with a test should be obtained *after* a discussion of risks and benefits. If things go wrong, you pay the price, which is why a risk/benefit analysis is always needed. Patients should use the term "risk/benefit analysis" verbatim when asking the doctor about the best way to approach an illness and not rely on the old "What would you do if you were me?" approach.

When will test results be available?

Ask for a time frame in which to expect your test results. If this information is not provided automatically, be sure to ask. You don't want to start waiting anxiously by the phone until they can actually be expected to call you. Remember, results of tests performed late in the week may not be available until the following week.

How will you be notified of the results?

Who will be responsible for reporting test results to you or your advocate? Often, the technician performing a scan will tell you that your doctor will be the one to call you, but that doesn't necessarily let you know when her department will provide the results to your doctor. It helps to know how your physician will receive the results—by phone, fax or mail. If it's by phone, you can assume it will be faster, and there will be an opportunity for one-on-one interaction, which is a great benefit to you. When the doctor can ask questions on the spot, he can obtain a more complete picture to pass on to you.

If you don't hear from your physician, always phone the office to check on your results. *Never* assume that "no news is good news." Whoever the designated hitter is, he ought to be qualified to answer any questions you have when he calls. If he is not able to answer them right then and there, ask for your physician to call you back. There is no reason for you to have unanswered questions about the test or its results after the final report is complete. You will also want to request a copy of your test results for your medical diary. Then read the report to be sure that it matches with what you were told over the phone. If you see any words or terms that strike you as less than perfectly normal, be sure to call your doctor back to ask about their meaning.

Are additional tests needed to confirm a diagnosis?

Are certain results inconclusive or conflicting or not a good "fit" with the clinical picture? If so, the tests may need to be repeated. Or additional ones will have to be ordered. As annoying as this can be, it's a lot better than a false result becoming the cornerstone of your treatment plan. An important last point is that if you have the tests reviewed by a second professional, it could actually reduce your need for additional tests.

What do my test results mean?

It is your responsibility to understand what information was gained from each test and to ask whether it will have any impact on your course of treatment. If numerical values are involved, ask if they are in the normal range. If they are not, find out how far out of range they are. For example, patients are often told, using vague language that their blood tests "are in an acceptable range" or "look better than yesterday." Even if blood test results have "improved," a lower number of white blood cells could leave you ripe for infection. Knowing that your white count is slightly reduced will make you all the more careful about washing your hands on a continual basis and being sure that your visitors aren't sick when they enter your room. Patients will be able to participate in meaningful discussions about their test results by asking a few basic questions.

Make the Most of Your Time with Your Physicians

Be organized

Have a pad and pen next to your bed at all times and write down your questions and concerns just as they come to mind when you're in the hospital. This will help you make the most effective use of the limited time you will have with a physician each day. If several doctors are consulting on your case, ask for their business card when they come in the room and jot notes on the back about who they are and what they said.

Have an advocate

For important consultations or treatment discussions, bring a friend or relative you trust who is not intimidated by the medical system. The advocate also needs to be easily accessible to you and your doctor. (A good friend who travels on business regularly or a mom with several young children won't be able to accommodate you, no matter how much they want to.) The person should also have her own transportation. If you are hospitalized, you may want to have an advocate present when your physician makes the daily rounds because she can take notes, help you voice questions and understand your treatment.

The "plan for care"

It is in your best interest to understand the daily treatment plan as well as the comprehensive recovery plan. A day in the life of a hospitalized patient can seem like a whirlwind. You are wheeled up and down endless hallways, poked and pecked at, examined by strangers, talked about as if you weren't in the room, pushed to your limit by a physical therapist, and told by nutritionists what you can and can't eat. It is easy to be overwhelmed by the many components of your care and lose sight of the overall picture and goals.

When it's time for daily rounds, try to be at the top of your game. Some hospitals are routinely conducting rounds right at the patient's bedside. This is when the day's plan for care is explained to you and when all your questions will be answered in layman's terms. It can be a big job to assimilate all this information because it is not something you are used to doing. This is why an advocate and a diary are invaluable; they help you stay focused on your treatment goals. Patients who understand each day's plan and how it helps to accomplish their treatment goals will be less anxious and much more motivated.

An appropriate amount of time with your physician

There are times when you need extra time to converse with your physicians. When scheduling office visits, let the staff know that you need additional time with the doctor and ask for an appointment when the doctor will not be rushed. Does your physician have an email address? If not, let her know that you are interested in this service and ask if it can be added to the practice. This is one way many patients have their questions answered without going through a lengthy office visit or playing phone tag all day. I have seen patients and their family members email their doctor right from the hospital —an extremely effective mode of communication.

Again I return to the question of rounds. When you're in the hospital, you need to know when they will be made so you can be ready for that crucial time with the doctor. It may only be for a few minutes, but it is the most important segment of the day. Find out if rounds are made everyday. Are they made on weekends? Since the house staff often conducts rounds, ask if your attending physician will be present. What will be his or her role in the daily plan for your care? For example, will he or she merely be reading your chart at the end of the day to see what their resident's have ordered for you? Or, will he or she be actively overseeing your progress and checking treatment plan updates as they happen? It is also important to realize that some hospitals are specifically including family members as part of the "team" during rounds. Ask the staff to include you or your advocate in their rounds and be sure that your advocate can be present at the designated time. Notify your nurse or patient relations representatives if you feel the need to schedule more time with your physician than rounds allow for.

Accessibility

How accessible are the physicians in charge of your care when you have questions, experience a complication, or simply need to inquire about changing your medication? Are patient care duties assigned on a rotating schedule, and if so, when does the schedule change? Who is actually writing the orders for your treatment, and how can you reach the person if concerns arise? Verify with the nurses that they are able to contact the doctor writing the orders at all times, including evenings and weekends.

After hours and on-call groups

Ask your physicians in advance how available they will be after hours and request that they review your case ahead of time, and if necessary, meet with you or your family. It is also vital to know is who will respond to inpatient emergencies during the day and what their training level is. Is there an attending physician to supervise interns and residents after hours?

Find out which doctors are included in your primary care physician's on-call group and what its size is. Do the doctors all know each other well and have similar styles of practicing medicine? An on-call group made up of 20 doctors (not uncommon in large group pediatric practices) will virtually assure that there will be a variety of styles and levels of aggressiveness when treating unfamiliar patients. Do the doctors in the group share the same specialty? If not, what other types of doctors are included? Are all the doctors in the group practicing medicine on a regular basis, or does it include doctors who are primarily researchers, in which case their hands-on experience will probably be limited.

Plan for Returning Home from the Hospital

It is frustrating to sit and wonder everyday if you are any closer to going home from the hospital. Of course, asking this too early in the game will probably result in the staff putting you off, but there is a point at which efforts by the patient can speed up the process.

Instead of passively waiting for a physician to update you, you can assume a proactive role by asking the simple question, "What needs to happen before I can go home?" Here are common examples of what you might hear:

- You need to be able to urinate so we can remove your catheter

- You have to be able to keep down solid foods

- You have to be without a fever for 24 hours

- You have to be able to manage your pain with oral medications and not IV meds

Patients who are given real, tangible goals will certainly be less frustrated. They will know exactly what conditions are keeping them in the hospital and which ones must change in order to be released. Anyone who visits someone in the hospital knows that the first topic of conversation is "How are you feeling?" followed closely by "When do they think you can go home?" The response I usually get goes something like this: "They don't tell me anything. I have no idea when I'm going to get out of here." When I hear this, I see a wasted opportunity to engage the patient as an ally in the quest to send a healed, healthy individual home where she belongs. Patients want to help expedite their release; they only need to be given the opportunity. What do they have to eat, how far do they have to walk, how soon do they to use the toilet themselves; tell patients this, and they'll be at the hospital's front doors waiting for their ride in no time.

Conclusion

Almost daily, our news media reports on astounding medical innovations, research and technology. And while these stories infuse us with a sense of pride and a general feeling of comfort and trust, the fact remains that there is a perilous side of healthcare. We have a system that can train medical teams to routinely perform complicated heart transplants, yet cannot ensure that the heart is placed in the correct patient every single time, with no exception. We have an industry that can unblock your coronary arteries without invasive surgery, use a gamma knife to treat a brain lesion and implant titanium joints that often function as well as the ones you were born with, and yet it loses tens of thousands of patients each year to *totally preventable* infections and errors.

Caring for and curing our bodies will always be inherently risky. That fact is undeniable. No one can ever guarantee that you will not encounter an unanticipated risk, a serious side-effect or an adverse outcome. What I can promise you, however, is that the action steps and advice in this book will help you combat the flaws in our medical system. They are realistic, achievable and could very well save your life or the life of someone you love.

Can you really accomplish the goals presented in this book? The answer is a resounding yes. The learning curve is not that steep – in fact, what you are really doing is modifying and expanding on skills you already possess. Asking the right questions, processing information and communicating effectively with others are tasks we all do every day. The challenge lies in being willing to investigate your condition by taking steps to educate yourself. In short, you are taking on the role of researcher and advocate.

I recently attended freshman orientation for my college-bound son. As I listened to the dean speak of the challenges facing college freshmen, I realized that they could just as easily be applied to healthcare recipients. Young adults are thrust into a new environment, they have to adapt quickly to new personal and professional relationships, and they must realize and accept the responsibility of making sure the college experience is everything they want it to be. It struck me that this is the exact mindset I am trying to convey to my readers. Perhaps medical patients need to see themselves as students standing at the brink of a new challenge in their lives and approach the situation with the focus and energy of a determined pupil.

To my readers and to all medical patients I would say this: the crucial first step is that you must see yourself as *worthy* and *capable* of being part of the healthcare team. What will give you the ability and the confidence to feel this way? Become an expert on your condition and learn the ins and outs of how the system works. Find out how to ask intelligent questions about your diagnosis and treatment and the right time to ask them. Hone your communication skills by interacting with your providers and be able to give them a concise and accurate accounting of your medications, medical history and current symptoms.

To the "system" and the powers behind it I would say this: Make your institution more patient-centered, meet every safety goal that the Joint Commission hands out, and recruit highly trained staff. In addition to that I would add the following: Have expectations of patients and their loved ones! Spend time educating them about their responsibilities and counsel them on the specific actions they can take to keep themselves safe. Ask patients to bring advocates with them to the hospital and to research their condition. Hand out medication lists for them to keep in their wallet. Ask them to write down their questions and concerns to share with staff. As soon as they are admitted to the hospital, tell them that they are a valued member of the healthcare team and you are counting on their invaluable input to improve the system for everyone. Invite patients to serve on ethics, safety and quality committees at your hospital. Encourage them to contact patient relations when they have questions. Inform them that they have a right to expect everyone who enters their room to wash their hands. Make them feel that they are well within their rights to expect safety and quality to be the overriding priority in their care. In short, give them the strategies, resources and the authority they need to become empowered patients.

We have to collectively stand at the forefront of a new era in health-care and say "The current health delivery system in this country—from the standpoint of the numbers of uninsured people, infection rates, medical error, staffing shortages, and medication mix-ups—is entirely unacceptable." We must be willing to lead the way in the quest for change because the system will only perform at its peak potential when we demand it. We have to be willing to work for healthcare reform and to challenge the political climate that continues to place it on the back burner.

To make a difference you don't need to be well-known, highly educated or influential. Every time I attend a patient safety meeting or connect with another advocate on a message board or website, I meet regular people who have become self-taught experts on such topics as surgical fires, medication errors, resident staffing laws or hospital-acquired infections. These were individuals who experienced first-hand the needless devastation of medical errors and decided to do something about it. Instead of giving in to anger or helplessness, they created websites to educate the public, gave lectures, lobbied legislators, joined recognized patient safety groups and wrote articles for their local papers. These people stand and bear witness to the fact that we can and must do more to keep patients safe.

Perhaps the most important thing they do is to share their stories, even though they are often painful and devastating, yet they do it anyway for the good of others. I hope this book inspires you to share *your* experiences, concerns and expectations with other patients, doctors, nurses, hospital administrators and your elected representatives. You can help ensure that we all receive the healthcare we deserve.

About the Author

Dr. Hallisy obtained her BS in Biological Science from the University of San Francisco in 1984 and a second Bachelor's degree in 1988 from the University of California at San Francisco in Dental Sciences. In 1988, Dr. Hallisy also received her Doctorate in Dental Surgery from the University of California at San Francisco School of Dentistry. Since then, she has been in continuous private practice in San Francisco, California.

Her second child, Katherine Eileen, was diagnosed at five months of age with bilateral retinoblastoma. The many recurrences of cancer and the subsequent treatments for the malignant and aggressive tumors began a 10-year immersion in our healthcare system.

Dr. Hallisy has worked with the California Nurses Association on the proposition 216 campaign for HMO reform. She has spoken at rallies with Ralph Nader and on camera for KRON Channel 4 in San Francisco. Dr. Hallisy provided testimony at San Francisco City Hall at the request of Senator Barbara Boxer to promote the passage of legislation for a Patients' Bill of Rights. She was the subject of a KGO TV news piece covering this event. In 2002, Dr. Hallisy spoke before the California State Senate on the issue of Futile Care policies. In 2006, Dr. Hallisy was a recipient of a scholarship from the National

Patient Safety Foundation to attend their annual national congress as a consumer advocate.

Please visit her website: Theempoweredpatient.com to tell us your stories and to alert others to any safety strategies that have worked for you.

Bibliography

Chapter One

…Ben Kolb…: Belkin, L. "How Can we Save the Next Victim?" *New York Times Magazine*. June 15, 1997; 28–70.

…Ben Kolb…: National Broadcasting Company. "Lessons from Ben: A Dateline Special (video). Chicago, Illinois. TeletechVideo, 2002. #NBDL020101.

…Lisa Smart…: Steinhauer, Jennifer. "Death in Surgery Reveals Troubled Practice and Lax Hospital." *The New York Times*. Nov. 15, 1998.

…Denise DeSoto…: Hernandez, Greg. "UC Agrees to Pay Huge Settlement in Malpractice Suit." *The Los Angeles Times*. June 21, 1998.

…Denise DeSoto…: Denise DeSoto, et al. v. University of California at Irvine Medical Center, etc. Superior Court of California. Case No. 73 10 46.

Chapter Two

A prototype for including patients in their care… *Joint Commission Resources*. Joint Commission perspectives on Patient Safety. Vol. 2, No. 8; Aug. 2002; 8–11(4).

"54% of house officers…": Wu, AW, Folkman, S, McPhee, SJ, Lo, B. "Do house officers learn from their mistakes?" *Journal of the American Medical Association*, 1991; 265: 2089–94.

"putting in a central line…": Volpp, KG, Grande, D. "Residents' suggestions for reducing errors in teaching hospitals." *New England Journal of Medicine*, Feb. 27, 2003; 348(9): 851–5.

...Marlene Joseph...: Statement of Leonard A. Joseph at the New York State Assembly Public Hearing: "The Disciplinary Process of Physicians and Physician Assistants." Jan. 31, 2002; New York, NY.
http://hometown.aol.com/pulse516/MarlenesStory.html.

...Dr. Karl Shipman...: Worland, Gayle. "Doctor's Orders." *Westword*. Mar. 25, 1999. http://www.westword.com/Issues/1999-03-25/news/feature2_print.html.

"Here is one tragic example." Rotstein, Gary. "No Place like Home: Nursing homes struggle with too few nurses, aides for growing elderly population." Post-Gazette.com, Sep. 22, 2002.
http://www.post-gazette.com/healthscience/20020922nursinghomes0922p1.asp.

...Rebecca Strunk...: Kunen, James. "The New Hands-Off Nursing."
The New York Times. Sep. 30, 1996.
http://www.time.com/time/magazine/printout/0,8816,985231,00.html.

Attorney General Pamela Carter...: American Nurses Association Press Release. "Nurses Voice Concerns about Patient Care in the Wake of Cost-cutting." Nov. 1, 1996. http://www.nursingworld.org/pressrel/1996/patsafe.htm.

Chapter Three

A 2001 study...: Wenzel, Richard P., Edmond, Michael B. "The Impact of Hospital-Acquired Bloodstream Infections." *Emerging Infectious Diseases.* Centers for Disease Control and Prevention. Mar.–Apr. 2001, Vol. 7, No. 2.

In 2000, the Institute of medicine reported that hospital infections ...: Institute of Medicine. *"To Err is Human: Building a Safer Health System."* Washington, D.C., National Academies Press, 1999.

...107,000 patient deaths a year...: Berens, Michael. "Unhealthy Hospitals." *Chicago Tribune*, July 21, 2002.

...hand washing at a teaching hospital...": Watanakunakorn, C, Wang, C, Hazy, J, "An observational study of hand washing and infection control practices by healthcare workers." *Infection Control and Hospital Epidemiology*, Nov. 1998; 19(11): 858–60.

"The April 1999 issue...": Kiely, P., BSN, Bacalis, L., BSN,RN,CIC, Hellinger,W. C. MD. "Interventions for Improving Hand Washing Compliance," *American Journal of Infection Control*, Apr. 1999, Vol 27, issue 2; 27(2): 208.

...Oklahoma City hospital had an outbreak of *Pseudomonas...*: Moolenaar RL, Crutcher JM, San Joaquin VH, Sewell LV, Hutwagner LC, Carson LA, Robison DA, Smithee LM, Jarvis, WR. "A prolonged outbreak of Pseudomonas aeruginosa in a neonatal intensive care unit: did staff fingernails play a role in disease transmission?" *Infection Control and Hospital Epidemiology.* Feb. 2000; 21(2): 77–9.

..."artificial or acrylic nails should not be worn"...(No author) "Acrylic fingernails pose infection control risk." *Journal of the American Dental Association.* 1999; 130: 1572–1574. http://www.jada.org/cgi/reprint/130/11/1573.pdf.

...15 defects per 1,000...: Department of Health and Human Services – Food and Drug Administration. "Medical Devices; Patient Examination and Surgeon's Gloves; Test Procedures and Acceptance Criteria." 21 CFR Part 800, Docket No. 03N–0056.

A study conducted at the Medical College of Georgia... Baker, Toni. "Study Explores Antibiotic Misuse." A Medical College of Georgia news release, Dec. 29, 2004. http://www.mcg.edu/news/2004NewsRel/wilde.html.

...fungal infections in a newborn ICU...": Chang, Huan J., M.D., Miller, Hilary L., M.D. Watkins, Nancy, R.N., M.P.H., et al, "An Epidemic of Malassezia Pachydermatic in an Intensive Care Nursery Associated with Colonization of Health Care Workers' Pet Dogs." *New England Journal of Medicine,* Mar. 12, 1998; 338(11): 706–11.

"A 1999 article by Pittet, et al.": Pittet, Didier, M.D., M.S., Dharan, Sasi, MT, Toureneau, Sylvie, R.N., Sauvan, Valerie, R.N., Perneger, Thomas v.,M.D., PhD, "Bacterial Contamination of the Hands of Hospital Staff during Routine Patient Care." *Archives of Internal Medicine,* Apr. 26, 1999, 159: 821–826.

...contaminated handle of a shared ear thermometer...": Porwancher, R., Sheth, A., Remphrey, S., Taylor, E., Hinkle, C., Zervos, M. "Epidemiological study of hospital-acquired infection with vancomycin-resistant Enterococcus faecium: possible transmission by an alectronic ear-probe thermometer." *Infection Control and Hospital Epidemiology,* 1997 Nov.; 18(11): 771–3.

...Pseudomonas aeruginosa...: Rutala, William A., PhD, MPH, Weber, David J., M.D., MPH. "The benefits of surface disinfection." *American Journal of Infection Control,* June 2004, 32(4): 226–231.

A 2001 article in Reuters Medical News... A. Neely, M. Orloff. "Survival of some medically important fungi on hospital fabrics and plastics." *Journal of Clinical Microbiology,* 2001, 39: 3360–3361.

A 1998 study published in the medical journal... Aintablian, N., Walpita, P., Sawyer, MH. "Detection of Bordetella pertussis and respiratory syncytial virus in the air samples from hospital rooms." *Infection Control and Hospital Epidemiology*, Dec. 1998; 19(12): 918–23.

...the antibiotic should be given at the right time...: Dale W. Bratzler, DO, MPH; Peter M. Houck, MD; Chesley Richards, MD, MPH; Lynn Steele, MS, CIC; E. Patchen Dellinger, MD; Donald E. Fry, MD; Claudia Wright, MS; Allen Ma, PhD; Karina Carr, RN; Lisa Red, MSHA. "Use of Antimicrobial Prophylaxis for Major Surgery." *Archives of Surgery*. 2005; 140: 174–182.

...the use of oxygen after surgery..: Greif, R., Akca, O., Kurz, A., Sessler, DI. "Supplemental Perioperative oxygen to reduce the incidence of surgical-wound infection. Outcomes Research Group. *New England Journal of Medicine*. 2000; 342(3): 161–167.

Keeping warm after surgery to reduce infection...Kurz, A. Sessler, DI., Lenhardt, R.: "Perioperative normothermia to reduce the incidence of surgical-wound infection and shorten hospitalization. Study of Wound-Infection and Temperature Group." *New England Journal of Medicine*. 1996; 334(19): 1209–1215.

VENTILATOR-ASSOCIATED PNEUMONIA SOURCES:

Institute for Healthcare Improvement. "What You Need to Know about Ventilator-Associated Pneumonia (VAP): *A Fact Sheet for Patients and their Family Members*." Accessed Jan. 2007 from http://www.ihi.org/IHI/Programs/Campaign/Campaign.htm.

National Quality Measures Clearinghouse. "Intensive care –ventilator-associated pneumonia (VAP) prevention: number of ventilator days where the patient's head of bed (HOB) is elevated equal to or greater than 30 degrees." The Joint Commission Intensive Care Unit Measure Set. www.qualitymeasures.arhq.gov, Feb. 2005.

Cavalcanti, Manuela, MD; Ferrer, Miquel, MD, PhD; Ferrer, Richard, MD; Morforte, Ramon, MD; Garnacho, Angel, MD; Torres, Antoni, MD, PhD. "Risk and Prognostic Factors of Ventilator-Associated Pneumonia in Trauma Patients." *Critical Care Medicine*. 2006; 34(4): 1067–1072. Copyright Lippincott Williams & Wilkins. http://www.medscape.com/viewarticle/528954.

HR Collard, S. Saint, MA Matthay. "Ventilator-Associated Pneumonia: An Evidence-Based Systematic Review." *Annals of Internal Medicine*. Vol. 138: 494–501. Mar. 18, 2003.

Guidelines for the Management of Adults with Hospital-Acquired, Ventilator-Associated and Healthcare-Associated Pneumonia. *AJRCCM*. 2005; 171: 388–416.

A story in the San Francisco Chronicle… Colliver, Victoria. "Recycled hip implants spell more suffering." *San Francisco Chronicle*, June 2, 2002.

Chapter Four

As many as 98,000…Institute of Medicine. *To Err is Human; Building a Safer Health System.* Washington, D.C., National Academies Press, 1999. Page 26.

One in every five deaths in medical ICU's… Tai, Dessmon Y.H., El-Bilbeisi, H., Tewari, S., Mascha, Edward J., Wiedermann Herbert P., Arroliga, Alejandro C. "A Study of Consecutive Autopsies in a Medical ICU: a comparison of clinical cause of death and autopsy diagnosis. *Chest.* 2001; 119: 530-6.

…Sturdy Memorial Hospital…Reuters Health. "Massachusetts hospital acknowledges 20 prostate biopsies misread between 1995 and 1997." Apr. 30, 1999. http://www.oncolink.com/resources/article.cfm.

TESTS RESULTS LOST: Smith, Peter C., MD, Araya-Guerra, Rodrigo, BA, Bublitz, Caroline, MS, Parnes, Bennett MD, Dickinson, L. Mariam, Ph.D, Van Vorst, Rebecca, BA, Westfall, John M. MD, MPH, Pace, Wilson D., MD. "Missing Clinical Information During Primary Care Visits." *JAMA*, 2005; 293: 565–571.

…a plane near Malaysia…ICAO Adrep Summary; Aviation Week & Space Technology 27.02.89 (24); Flight Int. 17-12.01.1990 (p.44)

…a third-year pediatric resident…Boodman, Sandra G. "Limited Experience, High Expectations." *Washington Post*, Mar. 23, 2001; page H01. http://washingtonpost.com/wp-dyn/health/A48834-2001Mar23.html

…physicians listen to their patients for an average of 23 seconds Marvel, M.K., Epstein, R.M., Flowers, K., Beckman, H.B. "Soliciting the Patient's Agenda; Have we Improved?" JAMA, Jan. 20, 1999; 281(3): 283–287.

…patients who are cared for by registered nurses… Needleman, Jack Ph.D., Buerhaus, Peter, Ph.D., Mattke, Soeren, M.D., M.P.H., Stewart, Maureen, B.A., Zelevinsky, Katya. "Nurse-Staffing Levels and the Quality of Care in Hospitals." NEJM, May 30, 2002; Vol. 346: 1715–1722.

…department of health and human services issued its final report on nurse staffing…Agency for Healthcare Research and Quality, Mar. 2004; No. 14. http:// www.arhq.gov

...the safe staffing law... California Nurses Association. Nov. 2005.
http://calnurses.org/nursing-practice/ratios/ratios_index.html

USA Today reported in April 2006 that wrong site surgery is increasing... : Davis, Robert. " 'Wrong site' surgeries on the rise." USA Today, Apr. 18, 2006.

Kwaan, Mary R., Studdert, D.M., Zinner, M.J., Gawande, A.A. "Incidence, Patterns, and Prevention of Wrong-Site Surgery." *Archives of Surgery*, Vol. 141, No. 4, April 2006. 353–357.

...the results of the largest study of surgical tools being left inside patients...: Gawande, Atul, M.D., M.P.H., Studdert, David M., LL.B., Sc.D., M.P.H., Orav, E.John, Ph.D., Brennan, Troyen A., M.D., J.D., M.P.H., Zinner, Michael J., M.D. "Risk Factors for Retained Instruments and Sponges after Surgery." NEJM, Jan. 16, 2003. Vol. 348: 229–235.

...the city of San Francisco settled a lawsuit...: Hartlaub, Peter. "S.F. settles suit over a painful pair of surgeries; towel, tubing left inside woman." *San Francisco Chronicle*. June 28, 2001.

"Be aware that there is new technology to help locate retained sponges...":Alex Macario, MD, MBA; Dean Morris, MBA; Sharon Morris, RN, BSN, CNOR. "Initial Clinical Evaluation of a Handheld Device for Detecting Retained Surgical Gauze Sponges Using Radiofrequency Identification Technology." Archives of Surgery. 2006; 141: 659–662.

...patients sustaining burns during MRI scans... Gosbee, John and DeRosier, Joe. "MR Hazard Summary." VA National Center for Patient Safety, Aug. 2001. http://www.patientsafety.gov/SafetyTopics/mrihazardsummary.html.

In 1993, Mrs. DeSoto was in a car accident... Denise De Soto et al v. University of California at Irvine Medical Center, etc. Superior Court of the State of California. Case No. 73 10 46.

BAR CODING: U.S. Department of Health and Human Services. "FDA Issues Bar Code Regulation." Feb. 25, 2004. http://www.fda.gov/oc/initiatives/barcode-sadr/fs-barcode.html.

...a two-month old child in Texas... Belkin, Lisa. "How Can we Save the Next Victim?" *The New York Times*, June 15, 1997.

MEDICATION ERRORS: Institute of Medicine. *To Err is Human; Building a Safer Health System*. Washington, D.C., National Academies Press, 1999.

...1.5 million medication errors...: Institute of Medicine. *Preventing Medication Errors*. Washington, D.C., National Academies Press, Dec. 2006.

...medication error rate of one per 6.8 admissions...: Institute of Medicine. *To Err is Human; Building a Safer Health System*. Washington, D.C., National Academies Press, 1999.

A 2004 study found an 11.1 percent error rate...Cimino, M.A., Kirschbaum, M.S., Brodsky, L., Shaha, S.H., Child Health Accountability Initiative. "Assessing medication prescribing errors in pediatric intensive care units." *Pediatric Critical Care Medicine*. Mar. 2004; 5(2): 124–32.

A study by Kozer et al...found prescribing errors...: Kozer, E., Scolnik, D., Macpherson, A., Keays, T., Shi, K., Luk, T., Koren, G. "Variables Associated With Medication Errors in Pediatric Emergency Medicine." *Pediatrics*. Oct. 2002; 110(4): 737–742.

...nurses at a Dallas hospital...: Winslow, E.H., Nestor, V.A., Davidoff, S.K., Thompson, P.G., Borum, J.C. "Legibility and completeness of physicians' handwritten medication orders." *Heart and Lung* 1997; 26: 158–64.

Error rates in the preparation and administration of medications... Barker, Kenneth N., PhD; Flynn, Elizabeth A., PhD; Pepper, Ginette A., PhD; Bates, David W., M.D., MSc; Mikeal, Robert L., PhD. "Medication Errors Observed in 36 Health Care Facilities."*Arch Intern Med*. 2002; 162: 1897–1903.

...10 most lethal medication errors... Argo, A.L., Cox, K.K., Kelly, W.N. "The ten most common lethal medication errors in hospital patients." Hospital Pharmacy, 2000; 35: 470–474.

...only 10 drugs account for over 60 percent... Winterstein, Almut G., Hatton, Randy C., Gonzalez-Rothi, Ricardo, Johns, Thomas E., Segal, Richard. "Identifying clinically significant preventable adverse drug events through a hospital's database of adverse drug reaction reports." *Am J Health-Syst Pharm*. 2002; 59: 1742–1749.

Research conducted by ISMP in 1999 found that only 44 percent of medication errors... Joint Commission Perspectives. Vol. 22, No. 3, Mar. 2002. 9–10(2)

...parents were told of medication errors... Ross, L.M., Wallace, J., Paton, J.Y., "Medication errors in a paediatric teaching hospital in the UK: five years operational experience." *Archives of Disease in Childhood*. 83(6): 492–496; Dec. 1, 2000.

...1.6 million-dollar malpractice award... Adams vs. Cooper Hospital, 684 A. 2d 506 (N.J. Super., 1996).

HOSPITAL BED SAFETY: U.S. Food and Drug Administration. "Hospital Bed Safety." Oct. 31, 2006. http://www.fda.gov/cdrh/beds/html.

In 2001, the FDA reported... "Panama Radiation Overdose Incidents." American Society for Therapeutic Radiology and Oncology. June 2001. http://www.astro.org/government_relations/capitol_hill_and_federal.html.

...four women died of asphyxiation... "Hazards of Nitrogen Asphyxiation." U.S. Chemical Society and Hazard Investigation Board Safety Bulletin. No. 2003-10-B. June 2003.

In 2001 a six-year old boy was killed...Rubenstein, Carin. "At a Hospital, 2 Instances When Things Went Wrong." *The New York Times*, Dec. 16, 2001.

...14.6 percent of Americans... Barclay, Laurie, M.D. (News Author) "Half of Americans May Meet DSM-IV Criteria for a Mental Disorder During Their Lifetime." Medscape Medical News. June 10, 2005. http://www.Medscape.com/viewarticle/506348 Original article: Kessler, R.C., Berglund, P.A., Demier, O., Jin, R., Wlaters, E.E. "Lifetime prevalence and age-of-onset distributions of DSM-IV disorders in the National Comorbidity Survey Replication (NCS-R). Archives of General Psychiatry, 2005 Jun; 62(6): 593–602. National Institute of Mental Health: http://nimh.nih.gov/publicat/numbers.cfm

...it is estimated that 7 percent of physicians are substance abusers... Cicala, Roger S., M.D. "Substance Abuse Among Physicians: What You Need to Know." *Hospital Physician*. July 2003; 39–46.

...staying awake for 24 hours... Dawson, D., Reid, K. "Fatigue, alcohol and performance impairment." *Nature*. 1997; 388–235.

Chapter Five

In a 1999 study of 6,000 patients... Kronz, Joseph D., Westra, William H., Epstein, Jonathan I. "Mandatory Second Opinion Surgical Pathology at a Large Referral Hospital." Cancer. Dec. 1, 1999; Vol. 86, No. 11; 2426–2435.

...two-year Rand Corporation study... McGlynn, Elizabeth A., Ph.D., Asch, Steven M., M.D., M.P.H., Adams, John, PhD., Keesey, Joan B.A., Hicks, Jennifer, M.P.H., Ph.D., DeCristofaro, Alison, M.P.H., Kerr, Eve A., M.D., M.P.H. "The Quality of Health Care Delivered to Adults in the United States." *New England Journal of Medicine.* June 26, 2003; Vol. 348: 2635–2645, No. 26.

...21 percent of eligible elderly patients receive beta blockers... Health Services Research on Aging: Building on Biomedical and Clinical Research. Translating Research Into Practice Fact Sheet. AHRQ Publication No. 00-P012, January 2000. Agency for Healthcare Research and Quality, Rockville, MD. http://www.arhq.gov/research/tripage.htm.

Fourteen years ago, Ms. Hillenbrand went to her doctor...Simpkinson, Anne A. "What Price Glory?" beliefnet, May 21, 2001. http://beliefnet.com/story/80/story_8043.html.

Lance Armstrong...asked to modify his treatment... Armstrong, Lance., Jenkins, Sally. *"It's Not About the Bike: My Journey Back to Life."* Berkley Trade; reissue edition. Sep. 4, 2001.

A ketogenic diet...Freeman, JM, Vining EP. "Seizures decrease rapidly after fasting: preliminary studies of the ketogenic diet." *Archives of Pediatrics & Adolescent Medicine*, 1999. 153 (9).

A shocking situation at a California Medical Center... CBS News, reported by Ed Bradley. "Unhealthy Diagnosis." July 27, 2003. http://www.cbsnews.com/stories/2003/07/17/60minutes/main563755.shtml.

In his book, *The Gift of Fear*...De Becker, Gavin. *The Gift of Fear*. Dell Publishing. May 11, 1999.

Chapter Six

A recent study by Thomas *et al*... Thomas, E.J., Sexton, J.B., Neilands, T.B., Frankel, A., Helmreich, R.L. "The effect of executive walk rounds on nurse safety climate attitudes: A randomized trial of clinical units." *BMC Health Serv Res.* 2005; 5:28.

...a heart procedure that was meant for another patient, *seventeen* contributing root causes were identified. Chassin, Mark R., M.D., MPP, MPH., Becher, Elise C. M.D., MA. "The Wrong Patient." *Annals of Internal Medicine*. June 4, 2002; Vol. 136, No. 11, 826–833.

...Johns Hopkins Hospital in 2004: Johns Hopkins University and Health System. "Spotlight: The Roots of Danger." Johns Hopkins Quality Update. April 2004.

...infection rates in many of the ICU's dropped to *zero*: Emery, Chris. "Simple measures reduce infections." *Baltimore Sun*. December 28, 2006. http://baltimoresun.com.news/health/bal-te.infection28dec28,0,7609251.story?coll=bal-home-headlines.

Chapter Seven

...new HIPAA rules explicitly permit...:Ross, Stephen E., M.D., Lin, Chen-Tin, M.D. "The Effects of Promoting Patient Access to Medical Records: A Review." *Journal of the American Medical Informatics Association.* 10: 129–138 (2003).

Chapter Eight

Johnson v. Kokemoor: Weber, Paul., JD. "Trends in the Duty of Informed Consent." EyeNet, November/December 1997. Ophthalmic Mutual Insurance Company. http://www.omic.com/resources/risk_man/deskref/medicaloffice/con....

Johnson V. Kokemoor: Supreme Court of Wisconsin. No. 93–3099, Mar. 20, 1996. 199 Wis.2d 615, 630, 545 N.W.2d 495, 501 (1996).

A 1996 survey conducted by the independent non-profit research agency ECRI: ECRI, "Managing the risks of sales representatives in the operating room: an HRC survey." *The Risk Management Reporter.* 1996; 15(5): 1, 3–7.

GHOST SURGERY: American College of Surgeons. "Statements on Principles." Section II, part D – The Operation – Responsibility of the Surgeon. Last Revised, Mar. 2004. http://www.facs.org/fellows_info/statements/stonprin.html.

Index

Printed in the United States
124789LV00002B/87/A

9 780615 177915